# Health Benefits of Pulses

Wendy J. Dahl
Editor

# Health Benefits of Pulses

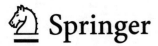 Springer

*Editor*
Wendy J. Dahl
Food Science and Human Nutrition Department
University of Florida
Gainesville, FL, USA

ISBN 978-3-030-12765-7          ISBN 978-3-030-12763-3   (eBook)
https://doi.org/10.1007/978-3-030-12763-3

This Springer imprint is published by the registered company Springer Nature Switzerland AG
The registered company address is: Gewerbestrasse 11, 6330 Cham, Switzerland

# Preface

Pulses, in the form of whole or split seed or flour, have been staple or subsistence foods in many parts of the world for thousands of years. The recent upsurge in interest in pulses and pulse ingredients, and plant protein more generally, in populations consuming mainly a so-called Western diet, has been driven by a variety of factors. These include consumer demand for high-protein foods prepared with non-animal-protein ingredients which are also non-soy, non-wheat, and non-GMO, the rise in veganism and vegetarianism, and anticipated health benefits associated with consumption of pulses, which are low in fat and rich in protein, lysine, dietary fiber, and resistant and slowly digestible starch and which contain a variety of micronutrients and bioactive compounds. From a wellness perspective, pulses seem right for the times in light of the growing prevalence in many countries of obesity and chronic, diet-related diseases such as hypertension, cardiovascular disease, and type 2 diabetes. The marketplace has responded to consumer interest in pulses with a flurry of new product introductions, which include pulse-cereal complementary foods and pulse-based meat substitutes and snack foods, along with an unprecedented level of commercial interest in wet and dry fractionation technologies and an upsurge in pulse production in North America and Asia, in particular. The increase in pulse production has been bolstered by the environmental and sustainability benefits stemming from the inclusion of pulses in crop rotations, in light of their nitrogen-fixing capability and consequent role in regenerative agriculture. This contributed volume includes chapters on the health benefits and metabolic impacts of pulse consumption and the role of pulses in solutions to malnutrition. Context is provided by chapters on future trends, global pulse consumption, and pulse processing and ingredient utilization. Anyone interested in the links between pulse consumption and improved health outcomes will find it a worthwhile read.

Gainesville, FL, USA                                                          Wendy J. Dahl

# Acknowledgments

The authors and editor would like to thank the following individuals for their contributions as reviewers: Tolunay Beker Aydemir PhD, Cornell University, Ithaca, New York; Julianne Curran PhD, Pulse Canada, Winnipeg, Manitoba, Canada; Asmaa Fatani MS, University of Florida, Gainesville, Florida, USA; Susan S. Percival PhD, University of Florida, Gainesville, Florida, USA; Anusha Samaranayaka PhD, POS Bio-Sciences, Saskatoon, Saskatchewan, Canada; Robert T. Tyler PhD, College of Agriculture and Bioresources, University of Saskatchewan, Saskatoon, Saskatchewan, Canada; and Yu Wang PhD, University of Florida, Gainesville, Florida, USA.

# Contents

# Contributors

**Melissa M. Alvarez** Food Science and Human Nutrition Department, University of Florida, Gainesville, FL, USA

**Getenesh Berhanu** College of Pharmacy and Nutrition, University of Saskatchewan, Saskatoon, SK, Canada

**Linda B. Bobroff** Department of Family, Youth, and Community Sciences, University of Florida, Gainesville, FL, USA

**Sam Buddemeyer** Food Science and Human Nutrition Department, University of Florida, Gainesville, FL, USA

**Fiona N. Byrne** Department of Nutrition & Dietetics, Cork University Hospital, Cork, Ireland

Department of Nephrology, Cork University Hospital, Cork, Ireland

HRB Clinical Research Facility, University College Cork, Cork, Ireland

**Mona S. Calvo** Retired, US Food and Drug Administration, Silver Spring, MD, USA

**Wendy J. Dahl** Food Science and Human Nutrition Department, University of Florida, Gainesville, FL, USA

**Claire Marie Fassett** Food Science and Human Nutrition Department, University of Florida, Gainesville, FL, USA

**Katherine Ford** College of Pharmacy and Nutrition, University of Saskatchewan, Saskatoon, SK, Canada

**Wendy M. Gans** Food Science and Human Nutrition Department, University of Florida, Gainesville, FL, USA

**Liwei Gu** Food Science and Human Nutrition Department, University of Florida, Gainesville, FL, USA

**Hiwot Abebe Haileslassie** College of Pharmacy and Nutrition, University of Saskatchewan, Saskatoon, SK, Canada

**Jeeyup (Jay) Han** Food Processing Development Centre, Alberta Agriculture and Forestry, Leduc, AB, Canada

**Carol J. Henry** College of Pharmacy and Nutrition, University of Saskatchewan, Saskatoon, SK, Canada

**Casey R. Johnson** Mayo Medical School, Rochester, MN, USA

**Kelly M. Johnston** Food Science and Human Nutrition Department, University of Florida, Gainesville, FL, USA

**Maryam Kazemi** Division of Nutritional Sciences, College of Human Ecology, Cornell University, Ithaca, NY, USA

**Shiv Kumar** Biodiversity and Integrated Gene Management Program, International Centre for Agricultural Research in the Dry Areas (ICARDA) Rabat-Institute, Rabat, Morocco

**Edda Lungu** Food Science and Human Nutrition Department, University of Florida, Gainesville, FL, USA

**Linda Malcolmson** LM FoodTech Solutions, Winnipeg, MB, Canada

**Meredith McSwain** Plant and Environmental Sciences, Clemson University, Clemson, SC, USA

**Adriana N. Mudryj** Department of Food and Human Nutritional Sciences, Faculty of Agricultural and Food Sciences, University of Manitoba, Winnipeg, MB, Canada

Ongomiizwin Research, Indigenous Institute of Health and Healing, Rady Faculty of Health Sciences, University of Manitoba, Winnipeg, MB, Canada

**Rachel L. Savelle** Food Science and Human Nutrition Department, University of Florida, Gainesville, FL, USA

**Dil Thavarajah** Plant and Environmental Sciences, Clemson University, Clemson, SC, USA

**Pushparajah Thavarajah** Plant and Environmental Sciences, Clemson University, Clemson, SC, USA

**Pooja N. Tolani** Food Science and Human Nutrition Department, University of Florida, Gainesville, FL, USA

**Susan J. Whiting** College of Pharmacy and Nutrition, University of Saskatchewan, Saskatoon, SK, Canada

**Yavuz Yagiz** Food Science and Human Nutrition Department, University of Florida, Gainesville, FL, USA

# Chapter 1
# Pulses, Global Health, and Sustainability: Future Trends

**Dil Thavarajah, Meredith McSwain, Casey R. Johnson, Shiv Kumar, and Pushparajah Thavarajah**

**Abstract** To feed the nine billion people who will be living on this planet by 2050 requires protein- and micronutrient-rich nutritious foods. In the late 1960s, the "Green Revolution" increased the production of cereals (rice, wheat, and maize) to combat global hunger by increasing caloric consumption. Today, however, millions of people around the world suffer from obesity, overweight, and micronutrient malnutrition. Health experts are now recommending a second revolution—a "greener" revolution—to provide not just food but more nutritious foods such as pulses: lentil, field pea, chickpea, and dry bean. Food legumes are a central part of the diet for many communities around the world, and therefore pulse crops could be a suitable whole food solution to combat obesity and micronutrient malnutrition. The objective of this chapter is to discuss the history of pulse crops, current production, nutritional promise, current breeding efforts at ICARDA (International Centre for Agricultural Research in the Dry Areas), and a successful case study whereby a Clemson University student created pulse-based community gardens ("Tiger Garden") to combat obesity and malnutrition.

**Keywords** Pulses · Biofortification · Sustainability · Micronutrient deficiencies · Low-digestible carbohydrates · Selenium · Antinutrients · Pulse breeding · Community gardens · Global health

D. Thavarajah (✉) · M. McSwain · P. Thavarajah
Plant and Environmental Sciences, Clemson University, Clemson, SC, USA
e-mail: dthavar@clemson.edu

C. R. Johnson
Mayo Medical School, Rochester, MN, USA

S. Kumar
Biodiversity and Integrated Gene Management Program, International Centre for Agricultural Research in the Dry Areas (ICARDA) Rabat-Institute, Rabat, Morocco

© Springer Nature Switzerland AG 2019
W. J. Dahl (ed.), *Health Benefits of Pulses*,
https://doi.org/10.1007/978-3-030-12763-3_1

## 1.1 Introduction

The "Green Revolution" of the 1960s to increase the production of cereals (rice, wheat, and maize) significantly decreased global hunger and energy malnutrition. Yet, more than one in seven people today still do not have access to nutritious food. The global hunger index (GHI) indicates world hunger has decreased by 27% since 2000, but 7 countries are still categorized as alarming, 44 as serious, and 24 as moderate in hunger (GHI 2017). Micronutrient malnutrition affects billions of people worldwide; 30% of the world's six billion people are iron (Fe) deficient, 17.3% are zinc (Zn) and iodine (I) deficient, and 15% are selenium (Se) deficient (WHO 2017; CDC 2017). Malnutrition has a global impact on individuals and societies, resulting in poor health, lower educational achievement, and a decreased work force, contributing to poverty, hunger, and social unrest. Micronutrient malnutrition is one of the most serious global health challenges faced by humankind, and is avoidable. Every human requires ~50 essential nutrients for general well-being and healthy living; however, the diets of more than two-thirds of the world's population lack one or more of these essential nutrients, leading to micronutrient malnutrition or "hidden hunger" (Copenhagen Consensus 2004; Bailey et al. 2015). Moreover, the world is now facing a new public health challenge: obesity, overweight, and related non-communicable diseases including heart disease, hypertension, type 2 diabetes, and cancer. Globally, 39% of men and 40% of women are overweight (BMI $\geq$ 25 kg/m$^2$) and 11% of men and 15% of women are obese (BMI $\geq$ 30 kg/m$^2$); in total, more than two billion adults are overweight and half a billion are obese (WHO 2017). The common saying "*what you eat in private, you wear in public*" is a good indication of the global awareness of obesity. Similar to hidden hunger, obesity also is a preventable health condition, and therefore populations need to make healthy food choices in their regular diets.

Healthy food choices are essential to combat obesity and micronutrient malnutrition. A healthy diet rich in dietary fiber including prebiotic carbohydrates, low in energy and glycemic response, moderate in protein, low in fat, and rich in micronutrients is recommended for body weight control as well as prevention of malnutrition (McCrory et al. 2010). Cereal-based diets are a good source of carbohydrates and can satisfy daily energy requirements, but do not provide daily requirements of protein and a range of micronutrients, including iron (Fe), zinc (Zn), vitamins A, C, and riboflavin, folates, selenium (Se), copper (Cu), calcium (Ca), and carotenoids. Protein and micronutrients are not only essential for general well-being but also are increasingly being recognized as important for disease prevention. Pulse crops (lentil, field pea, dry bean, and chickpea) have the potential to provide daily nutrient requirements in terms of dietary fiber, protein, and a range of micronutrients. Globally, pulse consumption has been declining as a result of economic transition, increasing household purchasing power, availability of low-cost fast foods, and a shift toward meat products (Thavarajah et al. 2016). For generations, Southeast Asians have regarded pulses as "*protein for the poor man*". Most Western populations are still not familiar with pulses, their nutritional benefits, and preparation methods as a result of the prevailing negative image of pulses as significant dietary components, which is based largely on misinformation about anti-nutritional factors, stomach bloating and discomfort, limited consumer appeal, taste, color, and longer cooking time. Despite these challenges, pulses offer a range of health benefits to mankind as well as increased global food and nutritional security; moreover, they offer ecological benefits in terms of nitrogen fixation and a low water and carbon footprint. Pulses are rich in protein and lysine, low in fat and energy, and contain a range of micronutrients, two to three times the levels in cereals, and the straw is a valued animal feed. Because of their vital nutritional role in human and soil health, farmers grow pulse crops with cereals, not only to meet food and nutritional security needs but also to maintain a favorable equilibrium in agricultural production systems.

## 1.2 History, Types of Pulses, and Current Production

The term "pulse" refers to grain legumes mainly used for human consumption or animal feed and is derived from the Latin word "*puls*", meaning thick soup, potage, or broth. More than a dozen pulse crops, *viz.,* adzuki bean (*Vigna angularis*), chickpea (*Cicer arietinum* L.), cluster bean (*Cyamopsis tetragonoloba L.*), common bean (*Phaseolus vulgaris* L.), cowpea (*Vigna unguiculata* L.), field pea (*Pisum sativum* L.), faba bean (*Vicia faba* L.), grass pea (*Lathyrus sativus* L.), hyacinth bean (*Dolichos lablab* L. Sweet), lentil (*Lens culinaris* Medikus), lima bean (*Phaseolus lunatus L.*), mungbean (*Vigna radiate* L.), pigeon pea (*Cajanus cajan* L. Millsp), tepari bean (*Phaseolus acutifolius* A. Gray), urd bean (*Vigna mungo* L Hepper), and vetches (*Vicia sativa* L.), are commonly grown in different parts of the world as components of subsistence farming in dry areas. These crops are the preferred choice among smallholder farmers (<5 ha), as they grow well under limited external inputs of nitrogen and water.

Globally, pulse crops occupy 81.8 million ha with a total global production of 74.7 million tonnes and average productivity of 913 kg/ha (Table 1.1). Dry bean contributes 34% to global pulse production, followed by chickpea (18%), field pea (14%), cowpea (7%), pigeon pea (6%), lentil (6%), and faba bean (5%). Globally, pulse production has increased 67% (30 million tonnes) over the past five decades (1964–2014) due to the combined impact of a production area increase of 12.08 million ha and a yield improvement as a result of pulse breeding efforts of 274 kg per ha. At the crop level, production increases over the last 50 years are most notable for dry bean (12.9 million tonnes) followed by cowpea (5.7 million tonnes), chickpea (5.6 million tonnes), lentil (3.8 million tonnes), and pigeon pea (2.7 million tonnes), while the greatest yield increase is observed for faba bean (859 kg/ha), followed by field pea (608 kg/ha), lentil (521 kg/ha), chickpea (376 kg/ha), dry bean (327 kg/ha), cowpea (263 kg/ha), and pigeon pea (79 kg/ha). During the same period, the area under faba bean and dry pea decreased considerably by 3.0 and 4.3 million ha, while cowpea, dry bean, pigeon pea, lentil, and chickpea have expanded

**Table 1.1** Area (million ha), production (million tonnes), and yield of pulse crops grown in 1961–1964 and 2011–2014 (FAOSTAT 2017)

| Pulse crop | Area | | Production | | Yield | | Gain/loss from 1961–1964 to 2011–2014 | | |
|---|---|---|---|---|---|---|---|---|---|
| | 1961–1964 | 2011–2014 | 1961–1964 | 2011–2014 | 1961–1964 | 2011–2014 | | | |
| | million ha | | million tonnes | | kg/ha | | Area | Production | Yield |
| Faba bean | 5.39 | 2.35 | 5.48 | 4.41 | 1016 | 1875 | −3.04 | −1.07 | 859 |
| Field pea | 11.12 | 6.86 | 10.85 | 10.87 | 976 | 1585 | −4.26 | 0.02 | 608 |
| Lentil | 1.66 | 4.39 | 0.92 | 4.73 | 556 | 1077 | 2.73 | 3.80 | 521 |
| Chickpea | 11.94 | 13.11 | 6.97 | 12.59 | 584 | 960 | 1.17 | 5.62 | 376 |
| Dry bean | 23.72 | 30.01 | 11.70 | 24.62 | 493 | 820 | 6.29 | 12.91 | 327 |
| Cowpea | 3.26 | 11.68 | 1.02 | 6.72 | 312 | 575 | 8.42 | 5.70 | 263 |
| Pigeon pea | 2.77 | 6.20 | 1.77 | 4.46 | 640 | 719 | 3.44 | 2.69 | 79 |
| Total | 69.72 | 81.80 | 44.59 | 74.67 | 639 | 913 | 12.08 | 30.08 | 273 |

into new niches due to robust demand from South Asia and Africa. Regional analysis of pulse production indicates that South Asia is the largest producer (39%) of pulses, followed by East Africa, North America, and other global production regions (Table 1.2). Major pulse producing countries in South Asia are India, Bangladesh, Nepal, and Pakistan. During the last five decades, pulse production in this region has increased substantially (up 56%), mainly due to a 17% increase in production area and a 33% increase in yield. Current estimates for area, production, and productivity of pulses in South Asia are 31.47 million ha, 20.37 million tonnes, and 647 kg/ha, respectively; chickpea is the major crop followed by dry bean, pigeon pea, lentil, and dry pea. East Africa now accounts for 11% of global production of pulses, with pulse crops planted on 9.53 million ha, annual production of 8.28 million tonnes, and an average yield of 869 kg/ha. Canada has emerged as the largest exporter of pulses to bridge the demand-supply gaps in South Asia, Southern Europe, North Africa, and West Asia.

## 1.3   Nutritional Promise

Malnutrition occurs as a result of protein, energy, and/or micronutrient deficiencies (including low bioavailability) in commonly eaten foods. Global micronutrient malnutrition has been addressed through food fortification, dietary supplementation, dietary diversification, and agronomic fortification of staple crops, but these approaches have had limited success (Combs 2001; Welch and Graham 2005). Inclusion of nutritionally superior pulse crops into local food systems has a significant impact by providing essential dietary requirements, especially in terms of protein and micronutrients (Thavarajah et al. 2014a, b). Pulses contain relatively high

**Table 1.2** Global regions of major pulse growing areas, production, and yield in 1964 and 2014 (FAOSTAT 2017)

| Region | Area 1964 | Area 2014 | Production 1964 | Production 2014 | Yield 1964 | Yield 2014 | Pulse crops | Country |
|---|---|---|---|---|---|---|---|---|
| | million ha | | million tonnes | | kg/ha | | | |
| South Asia | 26.86 | 31.47 | 13.09 | 20.37 | 487 | 647 | Chickpea, dry bean, pigeon pea, lentil | India |
| East Africa | 2.97 | 9.53 | 1.88 | 8.28 | 631 | 869 | Dry bean, faba bean, chickpea, lentil | Ethiopia |
| North America | 0.83 | 3.65 | 1.19 | 7.62 | 1435 | 2087 | Field pea, lentil, dry bean | Canada |
| Western Africa | 3.39 | 11.65 | 0.98 | 6.67 | 288 | 572 | Cowpea, dry bean | Nigeria |
| Southeast Asia | 1.20 | 5.02 | 0.82 | 6.52 | 681 | 1299 | Dry bean, pigeon pea, chickpea | Myanmar |
| East Asia | 10.21 | 2.95 | 10.00 | 4.68 | 979 | 1585 | Faba bean, dry bean, field pea | China |
| South America | 3.70 | 4.17 | 2.40 | 4.28 | 650 | 1025 | Dry bean, field pea, faba bean | Brazil |
| Eastern Europe | 10.79 | 2.42 | 8.02 | 3.80 | 743 | 1571 | Field pea, dry bean, chickpea | Russia |
| Australia | 0.04 | 1.87 | 0.05 | 2.45 | 1279 | 1314 | Field pea, chickpea, faba bean | Australia |
| Central America | 2.28 | 2.45 | 1.08 | 2.12 | 476 | 867 | Dry bean, chickpea, faba bean | Mexico |
| West Asia | 0.91 | 1.18 | 0.85 | 1.65 | 937 | 1402 | Chickpea, lentil, dry bean, faba bean | Turkey |
| Middle Africa | 0.59 | 2.29 | 0.29 | 1.40 | 496 | 610 | Dry bean, cowpea | Cameroon |
| Western Europe | 0.32 | 0.36 | 0.54 | 1.23 | 1651 | 3403 | Field pea, faba bean | France |
| North Africa | 0.88 | 1.06 | 0.78 | 1.12 | 887 | 1059 | Faba bean, dry bean, chickpea | Morocco |

concentrations of protein (~30%) and prebiotic carbohydrates, are low in fat, provide moderate energy, and are rich in essential micronutrients (Fe, Zn, and Se, folates, and carotenoids) (Bhatty 1988; Thavarajah et al. 2015a; Table 1.3). Most pulses contain low to moderate levels of phytate and polyphenolics, which may play major roles in antioxidant protection, energy regulation, kidney stone formation, and prevention of several cancers (McCrory et al. 2010). Biofortification of pulse crops through conventional breeding and modern biotechnology for target levels of micronutrients is possible, and is now recommended as an effective approach to mitigate global malnutrition (HarvestPlus 2017; Thavarajah et al. 2014a, b). As a result of current ICARDA biofortification research efforts, approximately 10–15 high bioavailability Fe and Zn pulse varieties are available for Southeast Asia and Africa.

**Table 1.3** Nutritional composition of common pulse crops grown in the USA

| Nutrient (units) | Lentil | Field pea | Chickpea |
|---|---|---|---|
| Moisture (%) | 1–12 | 1–13 | 1–7 |
| Protein (%) | 20–29 | 17–29 | 19–23 |
| Ash (%) | 1.8–3.3 | 2.1–2.8 | 2.4–3.1 |
| Total lipid (fat) (%) | 1–2 | 1–2 | 5–6 |
| Carbohydrate, by difference (%) | 60–63 | 60–63 | 60–63 |
| Total starch (%) | 40–70 | 36–75 | 44–65 |
| Energy (kcal/100 g) | 352 | 352 | 378 |
| Total prebiotic carbohydrates (g/100 g) | 12.3–14.1 | NA | NA |
| Resistant starch (g/100 g) | 5.5–9.3 | NA[a] | NA |
| Potassium, K (mg/100 g) | 545–1106 | 500–1008 | 780–1045 |
| Calcium, Ca (mg/100 g) | 45–54 | 50–80 | 16–99 |
| Magnesium, Mg (mg/kg) | 29–86 | 34–96 | 105–133 |
| Iron, Fe (mg/100 g) | 3.6–12.7 | 2.2–6.1 | 4.3–7.5 |
| Zinc, Zn (mg/100 g) | 2.3–6.5 | 1.9–4.0 | 2.6–4.5 |
| Selenium, Se (µg/100 g) | 20–83 | 7–58 | 35–68 |
| Ascorbic acid (mg/100 g) | 6.1–8.4 | 1.8 | 4.0 |
| Gallic acid (mg/100 g) | 0.3–0.4 | 3.1–3.4 | 3.2 |
| Chlorogenic acid (mg/100 g) | 1.0–2.0 | NA | NA |
| Folate[b] (µg/100 g) | 216–290 | 40–220 | 42–125 |
| Beta carotene (µg/100 g) | 110–313 | 19–1087 | 43–262 |
| Phytic acid (mg/100 g) | 240–440 | 270–320 | 58–136 |
| Fe bioavailability (ng/mg of protein) | 7.2–22 | NA | NA |

Data source: Thavarajah (2013), Sen Gupta et al. (2013), Johnson et al. (2013), and USDA (2017)
[a]*NA* not available
[b]Dietary folate equivalent

## 1.4 Low-Digestible Carbohydrates in Pulses

Carbohydrate components comprise about 60% of most pulse crops. These carbohydrates consist of starch, non-starch polysaccharides, lignin, oligosaccharides, disaccharides, monosaccharides, and sugar alcohols. Adding to the complexity, carbohydrates also are commonly categorized according to their nutritional properties. Dietary fiber often is considered "non-digestible" whereas other carbohydrates are considered "digestible". In reality, however, carbohydrates and fiber fall into a continuum of digestibility by enzymes in the human gastrointestinal (GI) tract. Glucose and sucrose, for example, exist at one end of the spectrum and are readily and completely digested by brush border enzymes and absorbed across the gut mucosa, whereas cellulose and hemicellulose are left almost completely undigested in most individuals. In the 1990s, Gibson and Roberfroid (1995) published the results of an important discovery regarding certain low-digestible carbohydrates, namely fructo-oligosaccharides (FOS). They found that FOS pass through the GI tract, avoid digestion by brush border enzymes, and pass into the colon where they are preferentially fermented by certain resident bacterial colonies. The products of these various fermentation processes afford health benefits to the host. The carbohydrate fractions have been termed "prebiotics." A revised definition for a prebiotic was published by the same authors in 2010: *"a selectively fermented ingredient that results in specific changes in the composition and/or activity of the gastrointestinal microbiota, thus conferring benefit(s) upon host health"* (Gibson et al. 2010).

More is known about the prebiotic carbohydrate profiles of lentil than of other pulse crops. The estimated concentration of prebiotic carbohydrates in lentil is approximately 12–14 g/100 g (Johnson et al. 2013, 2015a). Lentil contains (per 100 g) resistant starch (RS, 7.5 g), raffinose-family oligosaccharides (RFOs, 2.5 g raffinose plus stachyose, 1.6 g verbascose), FOS (0.06 g nystose), and sugar alcohols (SAs, 1.2 g sorbitol, 0.2 g mannitol). These low-digestible carbohydrate concentrations vary by region, country, and year produced (Johnson et al. 2013, 2015a). This variability in prebiotic concentrations may offer unique opportunities to maximize the nutritional potential of lentil and other pulse crops through plant breeding and locational sourcing. Moreover, cooking and cooling lentil leads to a twofold increase in RS concentration (Johnson et al. 2015b), providing additional opportunities for the food industry to optimize the nutritional properties of pulse-based food products.

Prebiotic carbohydrates exert their nutritional benefits through a variety of interesting physiologic mechanisms. Prebiotic carbohydrates can also be considered as "dietary fiber"; however, not all dietary fibers are prebiotics. This becomes important for understanding the mode of action as strictly prebiotic vs. related to dietary fiber. Beneficial functions of prebiotic carbohydrates are due to the actions common to most dietary fibers, including osmotic and pH changes in stool content, fecal bulking, and colonocyte proliferation as a result of increased "colonic food" from fermentation of these dietary fibers in the hindgut, the last of which results in increased colonic weight, length, and wall thickness (Kass et al. 1980). The combined actions of dietary fiber on hindgut microbiota result in enhanced fecal transit and the development of a more robust GI tract. For example, dietary fiber, including prebiotics, reduces the incidence of constipation, diarrhea, and GI infections and improves gut barrier functions. The cumulative effect of these processes over time protects against development and progression of a multitude of GI illnesses, including diverticulosis, diverticulitis, fecal impaction, and bowel obstruction (Aldoori et al. 1998; Voderholzer et al. 1997).

Oligosaccharides are considered the prototype for prebiotic phenomena: they are undigested by brush border enzymes but then are fermented in the hindgut, i.e., by *Bifidobacteria* and *Lactobacilli* spp., producing short-chain fatty acids (SCFAs) in the colonic lumen (Gibson and Roberfroid 1995). The most well-known examples of prebiotic oligosaccharides include FOS in chicory, Jerusalem artichoke, and allium vegetables (Gibson and Roberfroid 1995) as well as human milk oligosaccharides among exclusively breastfed infants (Gnoth et al. 2000; Walker 1998). Much remains a mystery regarding the exact mechanisms of how these beneficial bacteria, or their metabolites such as SCFAs, produce the various health benefits revealed in both animal studies and human trials. SCFAs, namely acetate, propionate, and butyrate, are small, volatile, carboxylic acids that are rapidly absorbed across the gut mucosa and are used as the primary energy source by colonocytes. These compounds act upon a multitude of protein receptors at the mucosal surface, provoking a range of physiologic and microbial responses involving hormones (Canfora et al. 2015; Hirasawa et al. 2005; Samuel et al. 2008), ion channels, transporters, immune cells, inflammatory and anti-inflammatory signals (Carnahan et al. 2014; Maslowski et al. 2009), and antimicrobial peptides (Schauber et al. 2003).

Receptor interactions with SCFAs at the gut mucosa modulate host inflammatory responses, thus moderating conditions such as obesity, inflammatory bowel disease, and other autoimmune disorders. SCFAs reduce the expression of TLR4 in colonocytes, a strong inducer of the inflammatory response (Isono et al. 2007). GPR43 receptors are activated by SCFAs, reducing lipolysis and free fatty acids in serum, and thereby reducing TLR activation and the ensuing inflammatory cascade (Maslowski et al. 2009). Treatment of neutrophils with propionate and acetate also suppresses the NF-κB and TNF-α inflammatory response induced by microbial lipopolysaccharide (Kiens et al. 2011). These data help explain why treatment of post-surgical diversion colitis with SCFA enemas improves remission of the disease (Harig et al. 1989). SCFAs also play a protective role against colorectal cancer via several mechanisms. SCFAs induce GPR43, which acts as a tumor suppressor in colonocytes. Furthermore, butyrate inhibits the genotoxic activity of several compounds in the intestinal lumen, creating a less genotoxic environment and protecting cell DNA (Wollowski et al. 2001). Finally, SCFAs act upon hormonal axes, controlling hunger and energy metabolism. SCFAs promote release of glucagon-like peptide (GLP)-1 from intestinal L cells, controlling satiety and metabolic hormone activity (Delzenne et al. 2007). Another satiety-promoting hormone induced by SCFAs, peptide YY (PYY), affects appetite and satiety by suppressing neuropeptide Y (NPY) and activating proopiomelanocortin (POMC) neurons in the hypothalamus (Canfora et al. 2015). Further promoting satiety, SCFAs inhibit ghrelin, which is a potent driver of the hunger response (Cani et al. 2004).

## 1.5 Minerals

Humans need approximately 16 essential minerals to maintain body physiological functions. These minerals are divided into two categories based on the quantity required by humans. Minerals required in large quantities (Ca, K, Mg, P, S, Cl, and Na) are known as macro-minerals, while those required in trace amounts (Fe, Zn, I, Se, Cu, Mn, F, Cr, and Mo) are known as micro-minerals. These two groups of minerals are equally important; the quantity needed in the body is not an indication of physiological or nutritional importance to human health. A balanced diet rich in different types of pulses can provide most of these essential minerals (Table 1.3). Recent biofortification efforts on pulse crops with highly bioavailable Fe, Zn, and Se have been able to supply the necessary daily dietary needs for vulnerable populations in Southeast Asia and Africa. For example, a 100-g serving of lentil provides a minimum of 50–100% of the recommended daily allowance (RDA) of most of these minerals (Thavarajah et al. 2007, 2008; Johnson et al. 2013). Similar promising results were reported for other pulses, including field pea, chickpea, and mung bean (Amarakoon et al. 2012; Thavarajah and Thavarajah 2012; Nair et al. 2013). Pulses are rich in most essential minerals (Table 1.3); however, their true mineral bioavailability depends on several factors including host physiology, gut microbiome, and the presence and availability of mineral absorption promoters and inhibitor compounds in the food matrix (e.g., ascorbic acid, carotenoids, prebiotic carbohydrates, phytate, and polyphenolic compounds). Several studies using in vitro digestion/Caco-2 cells and animal models indicate that mineral bioavailability is at least 10–30% for most pulses. A pilot study conducted in Sri Lanka with 33 mildly anemic children indicated the efficacy of a lentil diet to combat Fe deficiency anemia. The results clearly indicated that the group fed 50 g of split lentil per day for 2 months had significantly improved Fe status (Fig. 1.1). These results demonstrate the potential for consumption of lentil to improve the Fe nutritional status of anemic children in Sri Lanka and in other populations.

### 1.5.1   Selenium (Se)

Se is as essential to humans as are Fe, Zn, and vitamin A. Plants uptake Se from the soil and translocate it to the chloroplast where it seems to follow sulfur (S) and/or phosphorus (P) assimilation pathways (Pilon-Smits and Quinn 2010). Se and S are

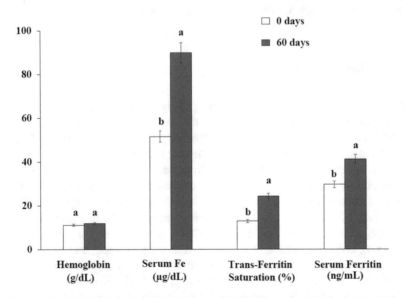

**Fig. 1.1** Blood analysis of mildly anemic children (n = 33) after 60 days on a lentil diet. Different letters above bars indicate significant differences at P < 0.05 between 0 and 60 days after treatment (n = 33)

similar in nature biochemically with respect to plant uptake and biotransformation. The human selenoproteome consists of 25 selenoproteins – NADPH-dependent flavoenzymes that function in intracellular redox regulation and catalyze the removal of iodine from the thyroid hormones. Selenoproteins consist of P (the major transport form), W (in muscle), and R (methionine sulfoxide reductase) (Kryukov et al. 2003). Two human diseases have been associated with severe endemic Se deficiency: Keshan disease (a cardiomyopathy) and Kashin-Beck disease (an osteoarthropathy). Each occurs in areas where the soil Se level is very low (<125 µg/kg) and locally produced grains contain <40 µg Se/kg (Combs 2001). Lentil Se biofortification is a feasible method to increase dietary Se intake for affected populations (Thavarajah et al. 2014a, b, 2015, 2017). The organic form of Se, selenomethionine (SeMet), is likely to have good human availability. Free SeMet is well utilized, being absorbed by the methionine transport system and then trans-selenated to SeCys, which is catabolized to selenide, the obligate form of Se incorporated into selenoproteins. Selenomethionine also is incorporated, as a methionine mimic, in general protein synthesis; this non-specific incorporation into proteins means that ingestion of SeMet supports significant tissue levels of Se. Because the same phenomenon occurs in plants, SeMet in lentil proteins might determine its bioavailability. A clinical nutrition trial in Sri Lanka (Thavarajah et al. 2011) clearly demonstrated that Se from lentil (727 µg Se per kg) was effective in raising blood Se concentrations in healthy Sri Lankan children. Children fed 50 g/day of lentil grown in North America had significantly higher blood Se concentrations 2 h after their meal (82 ppb) than children fed locally grown lentil (64 ppb). Thus, lentil that contains nutritionally significant amounts of bioavailable Se can make important contributions to public health, particularly in Southeast Asia.

## 1.5.2   Antinutrients

Pulses are not common in the diet of some populations mainly due to the perception of high levels of anti-nutritional compounds and intestinal discomfort or bloating experiences. Phytic acid, protease inhibitors and phenolic compounds are the major antinutritional compounds in pulses. Phytic acid reduces the bioavailability of minerals due to the chemical complexes of phytic acid and cations. Protease inhibitors reduce protein digestibility, and phenolic compounds complex with minerals and vitamins, thereby impacting their availability. However, these long-held notions are challenged by recent studies that indicate bioavailability is more complicated (Thavarajah et al. 2009). For example, phytic acid and inositol hexaphosphates, which are forms of phytates, were analyzed in the past using colorimetric procedures that returned crude total phosphate measurements and likely resulted in overestimation of true phytic acid levels (Raboy et al. 2017). However, new methods such as high-performance anion exchange chromatography with conductivity detection (HPAE-CD) separates inositol phosphate isomers and accurately determines concentrations based on the conductivities of these isomers (Talamond et al. 2000). For example, recent studies show lentil has very low levels of phytic acid

(Thavarajah et al. 2009), which contradicts older studies that indicated pulses were very high in phytates. Pulse breeding programs over the last three decades have focused on reducing antinutrients, including phytic acid and protease inhibitors, which has yielded varieties with naturally low levels of these compounds. Most pulses are pre-soaked and cooked before human consumption, during which time leaching, autolysis by endogenous enzymes, and thermal breakdown reduce the levels of phytates and protease inhibitors. However, it should be noted that more and more research is highlighting that phenolic compounds have considerable beneficial effects as antioxidants, play a role in defense against pathogenic microorganisms, and have potential anti-aging properties.

## 1.6  Pulse Breeding at ICARDA

The pulse improvement program at ICARDA is built upon the foundation of its vast germplasm collection and the use thereof to breed varieties better adapted to different agro-ecological conditions. ICARDA holds 38,000 accessions of chickpea, faba bean, lentil, field pea, and grass pea. Except for a few traits, sufficient variability for important economic traits has been identified in the existing germplasm. To increase the use of this germplasm in breeding programs, the Focused Identification of Germplasm Strategy (FIGS) has been adopted at ICARDA with robust geographical datasets. The strategy has proven successful for various adaptive traits such as tolerance to heat, drought, cold, and salt, as well as resistance to insect pests and diseases. Such FIGS sets for chickpea, lentil, and faba bean are now available to national research and extension system (NARS) partners for advanced breeding and genomic research. The ICARDA breeding program generally uses parents of diverse origin with the aim to combine traits contributing to yield, phenology, and adaptation to major biotic and abiotic stresses, along with market and nutritionally preferred traits. Following a selection-hybridization-selection cycle, ICARDA constructs new breeding lines to deliver to NARS partners in the form of international nurseries (IN). These nurseries comprise a range of genetically fixed materials and segregating populations to provide opportunities to NARS partners for selection. On the basis of phenological adaptation, agronomically desirable traits, resistance to prevailing stresses, nutritional quality aspects, and grower and consumer preferences, NARS partners identify and select promising lines/single plants for eventual release as varieties for commercial cultivation. Over 350 varieties of lentil (137), kabuli chickpea (162), faba bean (75), and grass pea (7) have been released for cultivation in target countries. During the last 10 years, NARS partners have released 85 varieties of these crops using ICARDA material (Fig. 1.2).

Efforts are underway at ICARDA to design varieties with appropriate growth habits and efficient source-sink relationships, as well as to restructure plants in accordance with environmental requirements and cropping systems. Introgression of unexplored genes from wild relatives has been effective in terms of broadening the genetic base of important traits such as yield and resistance to biotic and abiotic stresses in mandated crops. The present focus of the ICARDA breeding program is

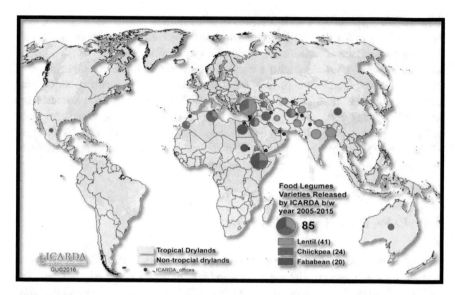

**Fig. 1.2** Improved varieties of food legumes released in different parts of the world using. ICARDA germplasm. (Reproduced with permission from Dr. Shiv Kumar, ICARDA, Morocco)

the development of improved varieties amenable to machine harvest with tolerance to herbicides, extra short duration Fe and Zn biofortified varieties for intensification and diversification of existing cropping systems, and climate smart varieties with tolerance to drought and heat. The ICARDA breeding program is pursuing a three-pronged strategy involving environment characterization using GIS tools, trait discovery using high-throughput phenotyping and genotyping platforms, and trait deployment through precision breeding tools in the desired agronomic background to enhance economic competitiveness and stability in performance of food legume crops under climate change. Biofortification, under the HarvestPlus Challenge Program of CGIAR, has led to lentil varieties enriched in Fe, Zn, and vitamin A. More than 1700 genotypes, including wild species, breeding lines, and released cultivars from about 20 countries, were analyzed for Fe and Zn levels (range: 43–132 mg/kg Fe, 22–90 mg/kg Zn). The high levels of Fe and Zn in wild accessions (ILWL74 and ILWL80) encouraged scientists to proceed further with genetic enhancement through cross breeding. Recently, a biofortified lentil variety, "Pusa Ageti", developed through cross breeding, was released in India.

## 1.7 A Place for Pulse Crops in Community Gardens

Community gardens are becoming an increasingly important component of both urban and suburban food systems, as the themes of sustainability, food security, health, and "returning to our roots" have gained popularity. This surge in popularity has been accelerated further by local, state, and federal programs that incentivize these health-based initiatives, i.e., locally grown food for healthy eating to combat obesity and malnutrition. Over the last 2 years, Clemson University's local legume and leafy vegetable garden project, also known as "Tiger Gardens", has been developed to combat micronutrient malnutrition and obesity in suburban South Carolina, USA, through hands-on academic enrichment at the grade school level (Plate 1.1). By creating raised-bed, community gardens at local elementary schools, the aim has been to experiment with and develop relevant curricula while working with local elementary schools to improve health and nutrition. The continual development of comprehensive guides in partnership with Clemson Cooperative Extension and a sustained presence in local garden chapters has allowed Clemson University undergraduate students to work toward improvement of local food security with an emphasis on nutritionally complete harvests.

Emphasis on the importance of pulse crops (field pea, sugar snap pea, faba bean, butter bean, and dry bean) has played a significant role in this community garden initiative by both directly and indirectly influencing curriculum design. Introduction to the diversity, impressive nutritional profile, and versatility of pulse crops has been important to the direct practical role students have had in the development of this

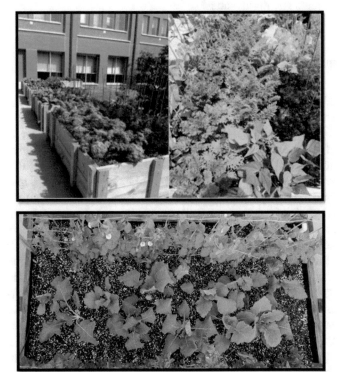

**Plate 1.1** Tiger Garden models using legumes and leafy greens. (Photo credits: Dil Thavarajah and Meredith Mcswain)

project through the planting and harvest of climatologically relevant pulse crops. This hands-on experience with the agricultural lifecycle of pulses has been key to improving understanding of an important and often neglected part of local, small-scale sustainable food systems. The practical aspects of this project also have been indirectly influenced by pulse crops through a focus on the growth of nutritionally complementary vegetable legume crops that may be easily supplemented with a variety of purchased pulses not suited for growth under community garden conditions. Furthermore, pulse crops are significantly represented in the educational aspects of the project, as exposure to the variety and nutritional depth of pulses is crucial for combating obesity and its linked non-communicable diseases through comprehensive education. The more technical side has been educational lessons on nutrient profiles of vegetables and the role these nutrients play in overall health. The importance of complete and balanced nutrition is a consistent theme throughout much of the accompanying curricular resources. Exposure to the dietary value of pulse crops has been assisted indirectly by the inclusion of recipes that incorporate pulses, even when they are not a primary part of the harvest in question. Overall, the synthesis of both practical hands-on gardening and nutritionally focused educational enrichment will serve to address more comprehensively the problems of obesity and micronutrient malnutrition, especially in food deserts where populations may be economically disadvantaged.

## 1.8   Closing Thoughts

Millions of people around the world are suffering from health issues related to diet. "Hidden hunger" and chronic, non-communicable diseases associated with obesity result in 36 million deaths globally each year, more than from all other causes combined. Furthermore, the global population continues to increase by more than 90 million people each year, with global food demand expected to double by 2050. With limited arable land, decreasing soil fertility, climate change, and declining water resources, food systems already are challenged with respect to providing sufficient nutrient-rich food to most global populations. Dependence on animal products is not an option for most of the developing world and is becoming more difficult in many developed countries. Therefore, novel ways to produce nutritious foods such as pulses are required to combat global micronutrient and calorie malnutrition. A range of pulse crops has the potential to provide sustainable food and nutritional solutions to improve human health. Integrated approaches to realize the potential of pulse crops in food systems requires a focus on human health outcomes. Crop yield is important, but equally so is nutritional quality to support human health. Finally, biofortification is a sustainable solution (whereas other fortification methods are not); therefore, further research on how to include a range of pulse crops in local food systems to combat global nutritional issues is warranted.

**Acknowledgements** The Pulse Quality and Nutrition program is supported by the Clemson University Seed Research (URGC); the International Centre for Agricultural Research in the Dry Areas (ICARDA), Rabat, Morocco; the American Pulse Association, WA, USA; the SC Department of Agriculture Specialty Crop Block Grant, SC, USA; and the USDA National Institute of Food and Agriculture – [Plant Health and Production and Plant Products: Plant Breeding for Agricultural Production] [grant no. 2018-67014-27621/project accession no. 1015284].

# References

Aldoori WH, Giovannucci EL, Rockett HRH et al (1998) A prospective study of dietary fiber types and symptomatic diverticular disease in men. J Nutr 128:714–719

Amarakoon D, Thavarajah D, McPhee K et al (2012) Iron-, zinc-, and magnesium-rich field peas (*Pisum sativum* L.) with naturally low phytic acid: a potential food-based solution to global micronutrient malnutrition. J Food Compos Anal 27:8–13

Bailey RL, West KP Jr, Black RE (2015) The epidemiology of global micronutrient deficiencies. Ann Nutr Metab 66:22–33

Bhatty RS (1988) Composition and quality of lentil (*Lens-Culinaris* Medik) – a review. Can Inst Food Sci Technol J 21:144–160

Canfora EE, Jocken JW, Blaak EE (2015) Short-chain fatty acids in control of body weight and insulin sensitivity. Nat Rev Endocrinol 11(10):577–591

Cani PD, Dewever C, Delzenne NM (2004) Inulin-type fructans modulate gastrointestinal peptides involved in appetite regulation (glucagon-like peptide-1 and ghrelin) in rats. Br J Nutr 92:521–526

Carnahan S, Balzer A, Panchal S et al (2014) Prebiotics in obesity. Panminerva Med 56:165–175

Center for Disease Control (2017) https://www.cdc.gov/immpact/micronutrients/index.html. Accessed 19 Nov 2017

Combs GF Jr (2001) Selenium in global food systems. Br J Nutr 85:517–547

Copenhagen Consensus (2004) http://www.copenhagenconsensus.com/copenhagen-consensus. Accessed 5 Jul 2017

Delzenne NM, Cani PD, Neyrinck AM (2007) Modulation of glucagon-like peptide 1 and energy metabolism by inulin and oligofructose: experimental data. J Nutr 137:2547S–2551S

FAOSTAT (2017) http://www.fao.org/faostat/en/#home. Accessed 1 Nov 2017

Gibson GR, Roberfroid MB (1995) Dietary modulation of the human colonic microbiota: introducing the concept of prebiotics. J Nutr 125:1401–1412

Gibson GR, Scott KP, Rastall RA et al (2010) Dietary prebiotics: current status and new definition. Food Sci Technol Bull Funct Foods 7:1–19

Global Hunger Index (2017) http://www.ifpri.org/topic/global-hunger-index. Accessed 19 Nov 2017

Gnoth MJ, Kunz C, Kinne-Saffran E et al (2000) Human milk oligosaccharides are minimally digested in vitro. J Nutr 130:3014–3020

Harig JM, Soergel KH, Komorowski RA et al (1989) Treatment of diversion colitis with short-chain-fatty acid irrigation. N Engl J Med 320:23–28

HarvestPlus   (2017)   http://www.harvestplus.org/biofortification-nutrition-revolution-now. Accessed 10 Nov 2017

Hirasawa A, Tsumaya K, Awaji T et al (2005) Free fatty acids regulate gut incretin glucagon-like peptide-1 secretion through GPR120. Nat Med 11:90–94

Isono A, Katsuno T, Sato T et al (2007) Clostridium butyricum TO-A culture supernatant downregulates TLR4 in human colonic epithelial cells. Dig Dis Sci 52:2963–2971

Johnson CR, Thavarajah D, Combs GF Jr et al (2013) Lentil (*Lens culinaris* L.): a prebiotic-rich whole food legume. Food Res Int 51:107–113

Johnson CR, Thavarajah D, Thavarajah P et al (2015a) A global survey of low-molecular weight carbohydrates in lentils. J Food Compos Anal 44:178–185

Johnson CR, Thavarajah D, Thavarajah P et al (2015b) Processing, cooking, and cooling affect prebiotic concentrations in lentil (*Lens culinaris* Medikus). J Food Compos Anal 38:106–111

Kass ML, Van Soest P, Pond W et al (1980) Utilization of dietary fiber from alfalfa by growing swine. I. Apparent digestibility of diet components in specific segments of the gastrointestinal tract. J Anim Sci 50:175–191

Kiens B, Alsted TJ, Jeppesen J (2011) Factors regulating fat oxidation in human skeletal muscle. Obes Rev 12:852–858

Kryukov GV, Castellano S, Novoselov SV et al (2003) Characterization of mammalian selenoproteomes. Science 300:1439–1433

Maslowski KM, Vieira AT, Ng A et al (2009) Regulation of inflammatory responses by gut microbiota and chemoattractant receptor GPR43. Nature 461:1282–1286

McCrory MA, Hamaker BR, Lovejoy JC et al (2010) Pulse consumption, satiety, and weight management. Adv Nutr 1:17–30

Nair RM, Yang RY, Easdown WJ et al (2013) Biofortification of mungbean (*Vigna radiata*) as a whole food to enhance human health. J Sci Food Agric 93:1805–1813

Pilon-Smits EAH, Quinn CF (2010) Selenium metabolism in plants. In: Hell R, Mendel RR (eds) Cell biology of metals and nutrients plant cell monographs 17. Springer, Berlin, pp 225–241

Raboy V, Johnson A, Bilyeu K et al (2017) Evaluation of simple and inexpensive high-throughput methods for phytic acid determination. J Am Oil Chem Soc 94:353–362

Samuel BS, Shaito A, Motoike T et al (2008) Effects of the gut microbiota on host adiposity are modulated by the short-chain fatty-acid binding G protein-coupled receptor, Gpr41. Proc Natl Acad Sci 105:16767–16772

Schauber J, Svanholm C, Termen S et al (2003) Expression of the cathelicidin LL-37 is modulated by short chain fatty acids in colonocytes: relevance of signalling pathways. Gut 52:735–741

Sen Gupta D, Thavarajah D, Knutson P et al (2013) Lentils (*Lens culinaris* L.), a rich source of folates. J Agric Food Chem 61:7794–7799

Talamond P, Doulbeau S, Rochette I et al (2000) Anion-exchange high-performance liquid chromatography with conductivity detection for the analysis of phytic acid in food. J Chromatogr A 871:7–12

Thavarajah D (2013) 2013 pulse quality survey. https://northernpulse.com/uploads/resources/944/2013-u-s%2D%2Dpulse-quality-survey-final.pdf. Accessed 24 Nov 2017

Thavarajah D, Thavarajah P (2012) Evaluation of chickpea (*Cicer arietinum* L.) micronutrient composition: biofortification opportunities to combat global micronutrient malnutrition. Food Res Int 49:99–104

Thavarajah D, Vandenberg A, George GN et al (2007) Chemical form of selenium in naturally selenium-rich lentils (*Lens culinaris* L.) from Saskatchewan. J Agric Food Chem 55:7337–7341

Thavarajah D, Ruszkowski J, Vandenberg A (2008) High potential for selenium biofortification of lentils (*Lens culinaris* L.). J Agric Food Chem 56:10747–10753

Thavarajah P, Thavarajah D, Vandenberg A (2009) Low phytic acid lentils (*Lens culinaris* L.): a potential solution for increased micronutrient bioavailability. J Agric Food Chem 57:9044–9049

Thavarajah D, Thavarajah P, Wejesuriya A et al (2011) The potential of lentil (*Lens culinaris* L.) as a whole food for increased selenium, iron, and zinc intake: preliminary results from a three year study. Euphytica 180:123–128

Thavarajah D, Thavarajah P, Gupta DS (2014a) Pulses biofortification in genomic era: multidisciplinary opportunities and challenges. In: Gupta S, Nadarajan N, Gupta D (eds) Legumes in the Omic era. Springer, New York

Thavarajah D, Thavarajah P, Combs G Jr (2014b) Selenium in lentils (*Lens culinaris* L.) and theoretical fortification strategies. In: Preedy VR (ed) Handbook of food fortification and health: from concepts to public health applications. King's College London, Springer, London

Thavarajah D, Johnson C, Mcgee R et al (2015a) Phenotyping nutritional and antinutritional traits. In: Kumar J, Pratap A, Kumar S (eds) Phenomics in crop plants: trends, options and limitations. Springer, India, New Delhi, pp 223–233

Thavarajah D, Thavarajah P, Vial E et al (2015) Will selenium increase lentil (*Lens culinaris* Medik) yield and seed quality? Front Plant Sci 6:356

Thavarajah D, Thavarajah P, Johnson CR et al (2016) Lentil (*Lens culinaris* Medikus): a whole food rich in prebiotic carbohydrates to combat global obesity. Agric Biol Sci. In: Goyal A (ed) Grain legumes. Intech. Print ISBN 978-953-51-2720-8

Thavarajah D, Abare A, Mapa I et al (2017) Selecting lentil accessions for global selenium biofortification. Plants 6:34

U.S. Department of Agriculture (2017) National nutrient database for standard reference release 28. https://ndb.nal.usda.gov/ndb/foods/show/4807?manu=&fgcd=&ds. Accessed 10 Nov 2017

Voderholzer WA, Schatke W, Mühldorfer BE et al (1997) Clinical response to dietary fiber treatment of chronic constipation. Am J Gastroenterol 92:95–98

Walker W (1998) Protective nutrients and bacterial colonization in the immature human gut. Adv Pediatr Infect Dis 46:353–382

Welch RM, Graham RD (2005) Agriculture: the real nexus for enhancing bioavailable micronutrients in food crops. J Trace Elem Med Biol 18:299–307

Wollowski I, Rechkemmer G, Pool-Zobel BL (2001) Protective role of probiotics and prebiotics in colon cancer. Am J Clin Nutr 73:451s–455s

World Health Organization (2017) http://www.who.int/nutrition/topics/ida/en/. Accessed 19 Nov 2017

# Chapter 2
# Pulse Consumption: A Global Perspective

Adriana N. Mudryj

**Abstract** Pulses (dry beans, dry peas, lentils and chickpeas) are nutrient dense foods that possess many beneficial effects. They are also among the most versatile and culturally diverse foods in the world, acting as a staple protein in certain countries. Although global pulse production has remained steady at around 40 million tonnes per year, in the Western world, consumption rates remain low in comparison to Asian and African markets, with Canada leading the global export of pulse crops. Future work directed at the long term benefits of pulse consumption on diet quality and disease reduction coupled with efforts targeted toward increasing global consumption rates are critical to reinforce the role of pulses in a healthy diet.

**Keywords** Pulses · Legume · Nutrient content · Pulse production · Pulse consumption · Dry bean · Chickpea · Lentil

## 2.1 Introduction

Pulses are among the most versatile and culturally diverse foods in the world, having a presence in diets around the globe for thousands of years. Historically, records of their cultivation, use and consumption have been discovered many places: from Peru and tombs in the Egyptian pyramids to small villages in Hungary and Switzerland (Leterme and Muñoz 2002). Due to their inexpensive nature, pulses earned the moniker of the 'poor man's meat', even recommended in medieval times by the Church as a substitute for meat during the Lenten fasting period. It also infers an association with poverty as far back as Ancient Greek times (Aykroyd quotes a line from the ancient Greek play *Plutus* by Aristophenes in which a character

A. N. Mudryj (✉)
Department of Food and Human Nutritional Sciences, Faculty of Agricultural and Food Sciences, University of Manitoba, Winnipeg, MB, Canada

Ongomiizwin Research, Indigenous Institute of Health and Healing, Rady Faculty of Health Sciences, University of Manitoba, Winnipeg, MB, Canada
e-mail: adriana.mudryj@umanitoba.ca

© Springer Nature Switzerland AG 2019
W. J. Dahl (ed.), *Health Benefits of Pulses*,
https://doi.org/10.1007/978-3-030-12763-3_2

remarks on a recent member of the newly wealthy "nouveau riche" *"Now he doesn't like lentils anymore"* (Aykroyd et al. 1964). Though this may have been uttered in jest thousands of years ago, even today there remains a positive association between meat consumption and one's income, with pulses remaining the prime source of protein primarily in countries where animal protein is far too expensive.

It is believed that the pea originated in the East, the lentil in the Middle East and the bean in areas of Central and South America (Leterme and Muñoz 2002). More locally, dishes such as the Quebecois-style pea soup, Southwestern and Mexican dishes and baked beans have played roles in North America's cuisine (Saskatchewan Pulse Growers 2010).

## 2.2   Nutritional Profile of Pulses

From a nutritional standpoint, pulses are a healthy food choice. Although characterized by a high carbohydrate content (~50 to 65%), they are slowly digested, placing them lower on the glycemic index (GI) scale than other carbohydrate-rich foods like rice, white bread or potatoes (McCrory et al. 2010; Ofuya and Akhidue 2005). They are high in fiber (Tosh and Yada 2010), and are an excellent source of micronutrients (Winham et al. 2008). Pulses are a rich source of iron and zinc, and although iron content is one nutrient that can vary greatly depending on the variety (e.g. white beans contain almost twice as much iron as black beans), a ½ cup serving of beans provides nearly 10% of one's daily recommendation (Patterson et al. 2009; Winham et al. 2008).

Research supporting the health and nutritional benefits of pulse consumption has been substantial (Anderson et al. 1999; Ofuya and Akhidue 2005; Papanikolaou and Fulgoni 2008). Emerging evidence has shown that a diet high in beans, peas, lentils and chickpeas can help protect against chronic diseases including cardiovascular disease, obesity and diabetes and contribute to overall good health (Health Canada 2008; Mudryj et al. 2014). Pulses are recommended as part of a healthful diet by both Canadian and American government agencies (Health Canada 2010; U.S. Department of Health and Human Services and U.S. Department of Agriculture n.d.). Both Canada's Food Guide to Healthy Eating (CFG) and the United States Department of Agriculture's (USDA) MyPlate nutrition guides group pulses in the meat and alternative group (Health Canada 2010; USDA 2017). Their high fiber content also allows them to be grouped within the vegetable group in the MyPlate guide (USDA 2017). The CFG currently recommends the consumption of pulses as good choices and the Dietary Guidelines for Americans suggest shifting food intake patterns to include at least 1.5 cups of cooked dry beans and peas per week. Additionally, it is hypothesized that the forthcoming overhaul of Canada's new Food Guide to Healthy Eating may place more focus on consuming plant-based proteins, like nuts, seeds, beans and lentils (Charlebois 2017).

## 2.3    Global Pulse Production and Consumption

Pulse production is highly concentrated. On a global scale, pulse production has remained steady at 40 million tonnes per year over the past decade (Faye 2007) with beans representing the largest percentage of global pulse production (46%), followed by peas (26%), chickpeas (21%) and lentils (10%) (Pulse Canada 2017). Currently, India is the largest importer of beans, peas and lentils: a country where pulses are an important source of protein for a largely vegetarian population (Food and Agricultural Organization 2016). Canada is the largest exporter of pulses, having developed a multi-billion-dollar pulse and special crops industry, followed by Australia, Myanmar, the United States and China (Food and Agricultural Organization 2016; Faye 2007).

The modern Canadian pulse industry began in the 1960s, with the production and subsequent export of field peas and lentils but did not play a significant economic role until nearly a decade later. During the 1970s, research work by Dr. Al Slinkard in Saskatchewan (the "heart" of Canada's pulse industry) was instrumental in helping previously unfamiliar crops such as lentils gain a wider acceptance by acquiring accessions from the United States Department of Agriculture's lentil collection and introducing them to a Canadian climate (Saskatchewan Pulse Growers 2010). The registration of herbicides allowed for new weed controlling methods, coupled with the overproduction of wheat, leading farmers to begin diversifying their crops to include beans, peas and lentils (Bekkering 2015; Saskatchewan Pulse Growers 2010). In the 1980s the industry expanded dramatically in response to international market demand, and in 2015 total production in Canada was a record 6 million tonnes worth nearly $4.2 billion (Pulse Canada 2017). Over the past two decades, Canada has become known as the world's largest exporter of lentils and dried peas, exporting nearly 75% of its production to over 150 countries around the world (Bekkering 2015; Pulse Canada 2017).

Outside of North America, pulses are important local food crops and a major source of protein, particularly in developing countries in Asia and Africa (Bekkering 2015; Faye 2007). Although the main amount of pulses consumed by Canadian consumers has increased over the past 25 years, it still remains low compared to countries where pulses are a dietary staple (Bekkering 2015). The Food and Agricultural Organization reports that consumption of pulses (on a per capita basis) has been slowly declining in developed and developing countries, reflecting not just fluctuating dietary habits and consumer preferences but also the failure of domestic production to keep pace with population growth in many countries (FAO 2016). In 2006, Statistics Canada estimated the domestic food consumption of beans and peas to be approximately 4.3 kg per person, or approximately 142,000 tonnes for all of Canada (Faye 2007; Statistics Canada 2007). Beans represented 75% of total sales, followed by peas (15%), lentils (9%) and chickpeas (4%) (Statistics Canada 2007). The Near East and North African regions of the globe are the only areas showing an increase in pulse consumption from 6.2 to 7.1 kg/person/year

(FAO 2016). Indeed, survey data shows that consumption in the Western world remains quite low, with only 7.9–13.1% of North Americans and Europeans consuming pulses on any given day (Eihusen and Albrecht 2007; Mitchell et al. 2009; Mudryj et al. 2012; Schneider 2002).

### 2.3.1   Europe

According to 1999 Food and Agricultural Organization data, the United Kingdom (UK) was the largest consumer of pulses in the European Union (EU), followed by Italy, Spain, Greece and Portugal (Schneider 2002). It is interesting to note that both amount of pulses as well as variety differentiates not only by region and culture, but also by socio-economic status, demographics and sometimes history. British troops during World War II consumed such large amounts of baked beans that Heinz required larger scale deliveries of high-quality, low-priced beans to meet the growing need. As a result, 80–100,000 tonnes of navy beans were imported from America, a trend which has carried on since then. Currently, UK bean processors import substantial quantities of beans from the U.S, Canada as well as China (Schneider 2002). In the UK, varieties such as chickpeas, faba beans and lentils are popular among African and Asian immigrants, while canned baked-beans are a staple in both "conventional" as well as vegetarian recipes (Schneider 2002). France, the largest field pea producer in Europe (although most of this production is designated to the animal-feed industry), has three main market sectors for its beans, lentils and chickpeas: those sold dry in grocery stores, stands or markets, canned pulses, and canned foods including pulses as an ingredient. French people 35–49 years of age are the most frequent purchasers of pulses, followed by those 50–64 years. Additionally, consumption is higher among lower socio-economic groups, household with four or more persons and in rural areas (Schneider 2002). Spain's small agricultural system means that it imports roughly 70% of its pulses from countries like Argentina, Mexico and North America (Schneider 2002). Schneider (2002) and Muzquiz (1997) describe the northern regions as typically being bean consumers, with expensive varieties being more popular in affluent urban areas. Lentils are mostly consumed in the southern regions of Spain, while chickpeas are popular in areas like Andalucia and Castilla y Leon, poorer areas of the country located in the south. Schneider describes Spain's uses characterized by local features: beans are often used in traditional dishes such as *fabada,* a meal consisting of pork and expensive, high quality white beans) and *cocido,* a chickpea and chorizo sausage dish. Beans are also a routine ingredient in soups, salads, and lentils are often popular as an accompaniment to sausage (Schneider 2002).

## 2.3.2   North America

Indeed, the pulse consumer profile varies according to each type of pulse, end-products and region in North America as well. In the U.S., a growing Hispanic population and changes to dietary awareness have been thought to have driven the per capita dry bean use. Using population data from the USDA's Continuing Survey of Food Intakes by Individuals, Lucier et al. (2000) found that although Hispanic Americans represented 11% of the total population, they accounted for 33% of all cooked dry edible bean consumption. This trend was also seen in work done by Mitchell et al. (2009) almost a decade later, with results showing that Hispanic and Mexican Americans were more likely to be pulse consumers than non-consumers. Low-income pulse consumers ate significantly more navy and pinto beans than those of a higher socio-economic standing. Additionally, black beans were consumed in substantially higher amounts in the southern states (Lucier et al. 2000). Previous research also suggests that education is a factor affecting pulse consumption, with a higher percentage of consumers having lower education (Lucier et al. 2000; Mitchell et al. 2009). While Lucier et al. (2000) observed that American men were more likely to be pulse consumers than women, Mitchell et al. (2009) did not detect any gender differences in consumption status.

Meanwhile, among Canadian pulse consumers, average pulse intake was highest in the province of New Brunswick (located on the east coast of the country), and lowest in Quebec, with the provinces of Ontario and British Columbia having the highest proportions of pulse consumers as residents (Fig. 2.1, Table 2.1) (Mudryj et al. 2012). Demographically, the highest proportion of consumers fell into the 51–70 year age bracket, similar to French trends (Mudryj et al. 2014; Schneider 2002). Pulse consumption in grams also differed between age groups, but not when expressed relative to caloric intake (Mudryj et al. 2014). Participants who identified themselves as Asian Canadian compared with Caucasian were 3.6 times more likely to be pulse consumers. As well, participants who identified themselves as being Arabic, Latin, African Canadian or of multiple cultural origins were 1.6 times more likely to be pulse consumers than Caucasians. However, gender, income, education level and community type (urban versus rural) were not found to be significant determinants of pulse intake (Fig. 2.2) (Mudryj et al. 2012) Tables 2.2 and 2.3.

The main sources of pulses in the adult Canadian diet were mung beans, Mexican or Hispanic mixed dishes, kidney beans, baked beans, bean soups and chili. These dishes made up 2/3 of the 22 dishes containing pulses in the Canadian diet mentioned in the 24-hour dietary recall using results from the Canadian Community Health Survey, Cycle 2.2 (CCHS 2.2) (Table 2.4). Pinto and refried beans represented only 1% of the pulse foods reported, while mung beans were the most popular pulse consumed in the dietary recall. This likely can be ascribed to the differences in the cultural mosaic of the U.S. and Canada. The American Hispanic population represents 16% of the U.S. population (United States Census Bureau 2017), while the same group represents only 1% of the Canadian population (Statistics Canada 2007). As Lucier and colleagues mention, approximately 1/3 of the beans consumed

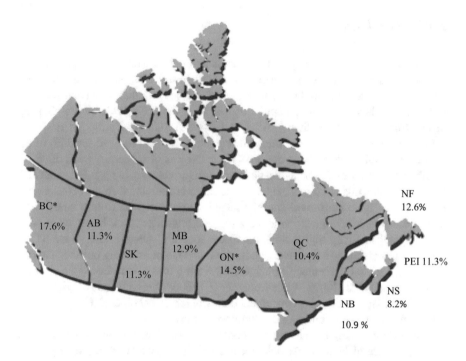

**Fig. 2.1** Geographic prevalence of pulse consumption in Canadian adults based on 1-day intakes from the Canadian Community Health Survey Cycle 2.2 (CCHS 2.2). BC: British Columbia, AB: Alberta, SK: Saskatchewan, MB: Manitoba, ON: Ontario, QC: Quebec, NB: New Brunswick, NS: Nova Scotia, PEI: Prince Edward Island, NF: Newfoundland
*p < 0.05, statistically significant in comparison with the province of Nova Scotia (the province with the lowest prevalence of consumption)

**Table 2.1** Mean pulse consumption (g) per province

|  | Total pulse (g) ± SE[a] | Total pulse (g) per 1000 kcal ± SE |
|---|---|---|
| Newfoundland and Labrador | 125.1 ± 20.8 | 47.7 ± 7.8 |
| Prince Edward Island | 109.7 ± 21.7 | 39.8 ± 4.7 |
| Nova Scotia | 124.3 ± 15.0 | 43.1 ± 5.8 |
| New Brunswick | 145.8 ± 34.9 | 35.7 ± 4.8 |
| Quebec | 82.6 ± 7.8 | 28.2 ± 3.0** |
| Ontario | 128.2 ± 23.4 | 40 ± 3.2 |
| Manitoba | 105.7 ± 12.4 | 35.4 ± 4.1 |
| Saskatchewan | 98.8 ± 21.4 | 33.0 ± 6.8 |
| Alberta | 96.0 ± 25.9 | 36.7 ± 12.0 |
| British Columbia | 111.4 ± 8.7 | 30.6 ± 8.7* |

According to 1 day 24 hour dietary recall of the CCHS 2.2 (2004) of Canadian Adults aged ≥19 year
*p < 0.05, significant when compared to Newfoundland and Labrador (the province with the highest consumption in g)
**p < 0.01, significant when compared to Newfoundland and Labrador (the province with the highest consumption in g)
[a]*SE* standard error

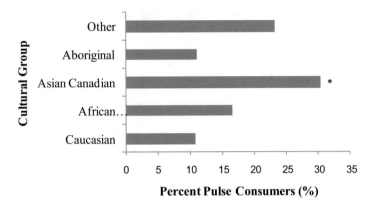

**Fig. 2.2** Cultural characteristic of pulse consumers in the Canadian adult population[1] (n = 20,156)
[1]According to 1 day 24-hour dietary recall of the CCHS 2.2 (2004) of Canadian Adults aged ≥19 years
*p < 0.05

**Table 2.2** Mean pulse consumption (g) by community setting

|         | Total pulse (g) ± SE[a] | Total pulse (g) per 1000 kcal ± SE |
|---------|--------------------------|--------------------------------------|
| Urban   | 72.2 ± 1.7               | 38.1 ± 1.0                           |
| Rural   | 77.8 ± 3.5               | 38.3 ± 1.6                           |

According to 1 day 24 hour dietary recall of the CCHS 2.2 (2004) of Canadian Adults aged ≥19 years
[a]*SE* standard error

**Table 2.3** Mean pulse consumption (g) per cultural group

|                                                      | Total pulse (g) ± SE[a] | Total pulse (g) per 1000 kcal ± SE |
|------------------------------------------------------|--------------------------|--------------------------------------|
| White                                                | 104.8 ± 5.1              | 34.5 ± 4.4                           |
| African Canadian, Latin, Arabic or Multiple origins  | 129.5 ± 34.4             | 48.0 ± 12.3                          |
| Asian                                                | 135.1 ± 37.4             | 35.2 ± 5.7                           |
| Aboriginal                                           | 90.9 ± 33.1              | 30.9 ± 15.3                          |
| Other                                                | 76.5 ± 44.9              | 40.5 ± 17.0                          |

According to 1 day 24 hour dietary recall of the CCHS 2.2 (2004) of Canadian Adults aged ≥19 years
[a]*SE* standard error

were by Hispanic Americans or consumed in areas such as California, Texas and Florida which have high Hispanic populations (Lucier et al. 2000). Conversely, the Asian population in Canada is approximately 10%, making up approximately 66% of Canada's visible minority population (Canadian Council on Social Development 2004), while Asian Americans represent less than 5% of the US population (United States Census Bureau 2017). The provinces with the highest proportion of Asians, Ontario and British Columbia, were also the two provinces found to contain the

**Table 2.4** Food sources of pulse products in the adult Canadian diet according to 1 day 24 hour dietary recall of the CCHS 2.2 (2004) of Canadian adults aged ≥19 years

| Food source | % of source reported |
| --- | --- |
| Mung beans | 18.2 |
| Mexican or other Hispanic dishes | 14.0 |
| Kidney beans[a] | 13.3 |
| Baked beans | 11.4 |
| Bean soups | 10.7 |
| Chili | 7.4 |
| Lentils | 5.3 |
| Chickpeas | 3.2 |
| Split peas | 3.0 |
| White beans | 2.9 |
| Hummus | 1.8 |
| Pinto beans | 1.3 |
| Refried beans | 1.3 |
| Black beans | 1.2 |
| Other bean sources[b] | <1 |

[a]Excluding chili
[b]Including rice with beans, navy beans, falafel, unspecified beans, bean dip, adzuki beans, winged beans, and noodles with beans, which each represent less than 1% of food sources reported

highest proportion of pulse consumers (Fig. 2.1) (Statistics Canada 2007), fitting in with the finding that Asian Canadians were found to be almost four times more likely to be pulse consumers. The prevalence of pulse consumption in the Canadian Asian population was also reflected in the predominance of the mung bean in the Canadian top consumed pulses list. Mung beans are grown in many Asian countries and are popular in many Asian dishes both as a sprouted form or cooked (Coffmann and Garciaj 1977).

Canadian adults who reported pulse consumption had enhanced micronutrient intake, especially in the highest quartile of intake (those who reported consumption at >290 g in any given day). The higher intakes of carbohydrate, protein and fiber among Canadian pulse consumers is likely due to these macronutrients being present in large amounts in pulses (Table 2.5) (Mudryj et al. 2012). Similarly, American adults who consumed approximately ½ c beans or peas per day had higher intakes of fiber, protein, folate, zinc, iron, and magnesium as well as lower intakes of saturated fat and total fat than non-consumers (Mitchell et al. 2009). Preliminary findings on younger respondents have also shown that children who consumed beans had significantly greater intakes of fiber, magnesium, and potassium than those who did not eat them (Fulgoni et al. 2006). These values are consistent with the nutrient profile of pulses.

However, Canadian pulse consumers had significantly lower intakes of vitamins $B_{12}$ and D. Pulse consumers also reported increased intakes of sodium compared to non-consumers, likely due to the high sodium content of canned beans. The high

**Table 2.5** Pulse amount and macronutrient, micronutrient and energy intakes per day for non-consumers and by quartiles of pulse consumption based on 1-day intakes from the Canadian Community Health Survey Cycle 2.2 (CCHS 2.2) 2004

| Quartiles of consumers | Non-consumers (n = 17,750) | Consumers (n = 2406) | | | |
|---|---|---|---|---|---|
| | | 1 | 2 | 3 | 4 |
| Intake category | | Mean ± SE | | | |
| Pulse amount (g) | 0 | 12.9±0.7 | 47.2±1.1 | 99.1±2.4 | 293.9±39.8 |
| Pulse per 1000 kcal | 0 | 6.1±1.2 | 22.8±1.2 | 38.5±5.3 | 75.6±3.4 |
| Food amount (g) | 3219±119 | 3540±441 | 3280±174 | 3315±139 | 3620±337 |
| Energy (kcal) | 2065±134 | 2279±318 | 2126±83 | 2299±133* | 2390±118** |
| Carbohydrate (g) | 253.1±15.6 | 279.8±38.1 | 255.8±11.6 | 285.5±16.1*** | 314.4±24.7*** |
| Carbohydrate per 1000 kcal (g) | 125.1±0.9 | 125.6±2.4 | 124.1±3.4 | 126.8±2.3 | 134.1±4.6† |
| Fiber(g) | 16.6±0.4 | 18.1±1.1 | 18.7±1.7 | 22.2±1.6*** | 30.7±2.2*** |
| Fiber per 1000 kcal (g) | 8.5±0.4 | 8.5±0.6 | 9.4±0.6 | 10.5±0.4*** | 13.8±0.7*** |
| Sugar (g) | 103.5±4.9 | 105.4±11.2 | 100.3±4.7 | 109.9±5.7 | 106.9±7.1 |
| Sugar per 1000 kcal (g) | 51.1±1.0 | 47.6±2.9 | 48.7±1.1 | 47.7±3.6 | 44.2±4.9 |
| Total fat (g) | 75.6±5.1 | 81.2±12.2 | 77.8±3.6 | 84.5±6.4* | 78.9±6.1 |
| Total fat per 1000 kcal (g) | 35.6±0.2 | 34.6±0.8 | 35.5±1.4 | 35.6±1.0 | 31.8±2.8 |
| Saturated fatty acid (g) | 24.8±2.0 | 24.7±3.1 | 22.8±1.6 | 26.2±2.3 | 23.6±2.2 |
| Saturated fat per 1000 kcal (g) | 11.7±0.2 | 10.6±0.5† | 10.3±0.5* | 10.9±0.4* | 9.4±1.1† |
| Monounsaturated fatty acid (g) | 30.3±2.1 | 32.9±5.3 | 32.1±1.5 | 34.6±2.6* | 32.9±2.2 |
| MUFA per 1000 kcal (g) | 14.1±0.1 | 14.0±0.4 | 14.6±0.6 | 14.6±0.5 | 13.2±1.3 |
| Polyunsaturated fatty acid (g) | 13.3±0.6 | 15.9±3.0 | 15.7±0.9 | 16.2±1.7* | 14.9±0.9 |
| PUFA per 1000 kcal (g) | 6.3±0.2 | 6.6±0.2 | 7.3±0.3 | 6.8±0.4 | 6.1±0.3 |
| Linoleic fatty acid | 10.6±0.4 | 12.9±2.9 | 12.4±0.7 | 12.8±1.4* | 11.7±0.8 |
| Linoleic fatty acid per 1000 kcal | 4.9±0.2 | 5.2±0.3 | 5.7±0.2 | 5.32±0.28 | 4.7±0.3 |
| Linolenic fatty acid | 1.8±0.1 | 2.3±0.3 | 2.4±0.2 | 2.5±0.3* | 2.6±0.3** |

(continued)

**Table 2.5** (continued)

| Quartiles of consumers | Non-consumers (n = 17,750) | Consumers (n = 2406) | | | |
|---|---|---|---|---|---|
| Intake category | | Mean ± SE | | | |
| | | 1 | 2 | 3 | 4 |
| Linolenic fatty acid per 1000 kcal | 0.9±0.0 | 1.0±0.1 | 1.1±0.1 | 1.1±0.1 | 1.0±0.1 |
| Cholesterol | 279.3±19.4 | 315.9±33.0† | 330.0±31.6* | 302.8±34.3 | 238.8±36.0 |
| Cholesterol per 1000 kcal | 138.7±2.3 | 139.8±10.6 | 150.1±9.1 | 130.6±10.4 | 103.5±12.7* |
| Protein | 84.5±5.3 | 94.3±12.6 | 91.9±4.5 | 94.9±7.9* | 100.7±6.7*** |
| Protein per 1000 kcal | 41.8±0.2 | 42.4±1.6 | 43.6±1.0† | 42.1±1.4 | 43.2±1.6 |
| Alcohol | 9.9±0.9 | 12.2±2.8 | 9.7±1.7 | 8.4±6.4 | 10.4±2.1 |
| Alcohol per 1000 kcal | 4.3±0.3 | 4.7±0.9 | 3.8±0.6 | 3.4±1.4 | 4.0±0.7 |
| Carbohydrate (% kcal) | 49.1±0.3 | 49.4±0.9 | 48.7±1.4 | 49.7±0.9 | 52.4±1.9 |
| Fat (% kcal) | 31.5±0.1 | 30.6±0.7 | 31.5±1.2 | 31.4±0.9* | 28.0±2.5 |
| Saturated fatty acid (% kcal) | 10.3±0.2 | 9.4±0.4† | 9.1±0.4* | 9.7±0.4* | 8.3±1.0† |
| Monounsaturated fatty acid (% kcal) | 12.5±0.1 | 12.4±0.4 | 12.9±0.5 | 12.9±0.4 | 11.6±1.1 |
| Polyunsaturated fatty acid (% kcal) | 5.5±0.2 | 5.8±0.2 | 6.5±0.3*** | 6.0±0.3 | 5.3±0.3 |
| Linoleic fatty acid (%kcal) | 4.4±0.1 | 4.6±0.3 | 5.1±0.2** | 4.7±0.3 | 4.2±0.3 |
| Linolenic fatty acid (%kcal) | 0.8±0.0 | 0.9±0.1* | 1.0±0.1** | 1.0±0.1 | 0.9±0.1 |
| Protein (%kcal) | 16.5±0.1 | 16.7±0.5 | 17.2±0.4† | 16.5±0.6 | 16.9±0.6 |
| Alcohol (%kcal) | 2.9±0.2 | 3.3±0.6 | 2.6±0.4 | 2.3±0.9 | 2.7±0.5 |
| Vitamin A | 696.4±58.9 | 695.5±109.8 | 750.9±73.3 | 755.8±95.6 | 643.9±57.4 |
| Vitamin A per 1000 kcal | 359.7±10.9 | 328.4±57.2 | 373.4±54.8 | 339.0±30.4 | 278.8±33.5† |
| Vitamin D | 5.6±0.1 | 6.0±0.8 | 6.0±1.0 | 6.3±1.5 | 4.6±0.4* |
| Vitamin D per 1000 kcal | 2.8±0.2 | 2.7±0.3 | 2.9±0.4 | 2.7±0.9 | 2.0±0.2*** |
| Vitamin C | 126.1±7.9 | 142.5±23.9 | 140.8±18.3 | 135.1±9.5 | 135.2±13.6 |
| Vitamin C per 1000 kcal | 66.3±1.3 | 68.8±14.4 | 67.8±5.6 | 61.3±3.9 | 58.3±9.9 |

| | | | | | |
|---|---|---|---|---|---|
| Thiamin | 1.7±0.1 | 1.8±0.3 | 1.7±0.1 | 1.9±0.2* | 1.9±0.3 |
| Thiamin per 1000 kcal | 0.9±0.0 | 0.8±0.0 | 0.8±0.0 | 0.8±0.0 | 0.8±0.1 |
| Riboflavin | 1.9±0.1 | 2.1±0.3 | 1.9±0.1 | 2.1±0.1† | 2.0±0.1 |
| Riboflavin per 1000 kcal | 1.0±0.0 | 0.9±0.0 | 1.0±0.0 | 0.9±0.0 | 0.8±0.0** |
| Niacin | 39.6±2.5 | 43.3±5.8 | 42.7±2.0 | 43.1±2.7* | 43.9±2.3 |
| Niacin per 1000 kcal | 19.7±0.1 | 19.7±0.6 | 20.6±0.5 | 19.0±0.5 | 19.0±0.5 |
| Vitamin B6 | 1.8±0.1 | 2.1±0.3 | 2.0±0.1 | 2.1±0.1† | 2.1±0.1** |
| Vitamin B6 per 1000 kcal | 0.9±0.0 | 0.9±0.0 | 1.0±0.1 | 1.0±0.1 | 0.9±0.0 |
| Vitamin B12 | 4.1±0.3 | 5.2±0.7 | 4.9±0.7 | 4.2±0.9 | 3.8±0.3* |
| Vitamin B12 per 1000 kcal | 2.2±0.1 | 2.2±0.3 | 2.4±0.6 | 1.9±0.6 | 1.6±0.2** |
| Naturally occurring folate | 226.9±12.5 | 250.2±30.7 | 250.0±10.3† | 295.9±40.7* | 423.6±69.1*** |
| Nat. Occurring Folate per 1000 kcal | 118.5±1.4 | 116.6±6.4 | 125.3±5.26 | 140.1±13.2† | 186.7±20.7*** |
| Folic Acid | 119.8±19.0 | 157.3±43.4 | 130.2±28.0 | 139.0±32.1 | 133.2±20.7 |
| Folic Acid per 1000 kcal | 58.5±5.8 | 67.9±10.1† | 59.7±9.8 | 58.9±7.8 | 56.3±8.5 |
| Folate (from food in dietary folate equiv.) | 452.9±34.1 | 470.3±66.6 | 450.0±16.1 | 540.9±80.3† | 655.9±59.0*** |
| Folate per 1000 kcal | 228.8±3.7 | 216.1±6.3 | 217.7±9.9 | 240.8±16.3 | 288.95±17.0*** |
| Folacin | 352.3±31.1 | 417.1±76.4 | 384.8±31.4** | 438.4±67.4* | 563.2±88.5*** |
| Folacin per 1000 kcal | 179.9±6.6 | 189.8±9.6† | 187.6±9.2 | 200.6±17.7 | 245.5±28.5** |
| Calcium | 865.4±62.3 | 884.5±93.5 | 748.4±52.5 | 937.11±69.8 | 953.8±92.9† |
| Calcium per 1000 kcal | 431.9±4.1 | 404.6±18.9 | 369.5±16.0*** | 416.4±15.8 | 401.8±26.1 |
| Phosphorus | 1329.7±63.1 | 1453.8±186.9 | 1352.4±61.8 | 1497.3±84.4** | 1597.4±107.9*** |
| Phosphorus per 1000 kcal | 659.5±11.4 | 649.7±17.8 | 657.4±18.9 | 670.7±19.1 | 687.0±25.0 |
| Magnesium | 322.5±14.2 | 358.9±45.6 | 339.1±14.8 | 374.6±17.1*** | 438.1±39.5*** |
| Magnesium per 1000 kcal | 165.9±4.5 | 166.0±3.7 | 171.1±5.5 | 174.7±4.8† | 191.5±9.7† |
| Iron | 13.9±0.7 | 14.8±1.6 | 14.1±0.5 | 16.0±0.7*** | 18.7±0.8*** |
| Iron per 1000 kcal | 7.0±0.1 | 6.8±0.2 | 7.0±0.2 | 7.2±0.4 | 8.3±0.3*** |

(continued)

**Table 2.5** (continued)

| Quartiles of consumers | Non-consumers (n = 17,750) | Consumers (n = 2406) | | | |
| --- | --- | --- | --- | --- | --- |
| | | 1 | 2 | 3 | 4 |
| Intake category | | Mean ± SE | | | |
| Zinc | 11.2±0.6 | 12.5±2.0 | 11.8±0.8 | 12.7±0.7** | 14.3±0.6*** |
| Zinc per 1000 kcal | 5.5±0.1 | 5.6±0.3 | 5.7±0.2 | 5.7±0.2 | 6.2±0.2*** |
| Sodium | 3050.2±169.6 | 3320.0±412.0 | 3368.9±141.2† | 3580.9±202.9† | 3987.6±250.4* |
| Sodium per 1000 kcal | 1522.1±32.6 | 1503.4±39.5 | 1613.4±57.7† | 1584.08±122.4 | 1720.8±143.2† |
| Potassium | 3074.2±93.5 | 3350.8±438.4 | 3191.5±160.0 | 3475.95±133.4 | 3926.5±152.5 |
| Potassium per 1000 kcal | 1583.8±56.4 | 1564.1±40.5 | 1597.3±86.8 | 1607.6±62.7 | 1707.8±66.2** |

*p <0.05, statistically significant in comparison with the non-consumer group
**p <0.01, statistically significant in comparison with the non-consumer group
***p<0.001, statistically significant in comparison with the non-consumer group
†approaching significance (p value between 0.05 and 0.1)

sodium "brine" that accompanies most canned pulses likely contributes to this as well as the most frequently consumed foods that contain pulses, such as chili or Mexican dishes (Mitchell et al. 2009; Mudryj et al. 2012). As well, foods such as hummus, which vary greatly in sodium content depending on commercial type, may influence sodium intake due to the addition of sodium chloride used in preparation (Al-Kanhal et al. 1998). Cooked dry beans are more energy-dense, providing more protein, fiber, iron, potassium and magnesium and less sodium per gram than their canned alternatives ($P < 0.05$). Additionally, canned beans that are drained contain significantly more energy than un-drained canned beans, as well as more total carbohydrate, protein, fiber, iron, potassium, folate, magnesium, zinc and copper (Zanovec et al. 2011). Draining and rinsing of canned pulses is an effective means of reducing sodium content of canned beans: draining beans removes 36% of the sodium (from 503 to 321 mg/serving), while both draining and rinsing removes, on average, 41% of the sodium (503–295 mg/serving, respectively) (Duyff et al. 2011; Zanovec et al. 2011).

Overall energy intake was higher in pulse consumers, a finding consistent with the US population analysis (Mitchell et al. 2009). It would be expected that this higher energy intake by pulse consumers would be associated with an increased body mass. However, although mean BMI was higher in pulse consumers ($28.0 \pm 0.75$ and $27.3 \pm 0.11$, respectively), this difference was not statistically significant. This trend is in contrast to other findings which suggest that high fiber foods such as pulses lead to an increased feeling of fullness and may lead to a healthier body weight when eaten at higher amounts (Papanikolaou and Fulgoni 2008). The reason for this apparent discrepancy cannot be determined from the survey data, but it may be that other foods consumed along with pulses may counteract the expected satiating effects of high fiber pulses. The effect of pulse consumption on body weight also may be confounded by the fact that a large proportion of Canadians are in the overweight BMI category (Health Canada 2010).

## 2.4  Factors Influencing Pulse Consumption

Although literature is lacking on the reasons why intake of pulses is low (particularly in Western societies), there appear to be a few key causes. These include unpleasant gastrointestinal side effects, constraints on cooking, and taste levels. In their article examining pulse consumption in Latin America, Leterme and Muñoz (2002) cite length of cooking as a top influence in abstaining from pulses (particularly in areas where pressure cookers are not commonplace), followed by taste aversion and flatulence. Eihusen and Albrecht (2007) examined pulse intake in American females ages 19–45 and listed various reasons as to why the women studied did not consume beans. These included taste (21.8%), lengthy cooking time (20%), uncomfortable gastrointestinal side effects (14.6%) and availability (5.5%) as well as combinations of these factors. It is interesting to note that when these authors examined reasons why women include dry beans in their diet, taste was also a factor (30.3%), followed by nutritional value (15.9%) and tradition (8.3%).

## 2.5 Conclusions

Currently in the Western world, pulse consumption levels are fairly low, indicating a potential for pulses to make a significant contribution to maintaining overall health and preventing disease. Traditionally, North American diets have not featured large-scale pulse consumption due to ease and access to other protein sources, such as meat. However, the low cost of pulses represents an important factor Recently a massive global marketing effort crowned 2016 as "The International Year of Pulses", with the goal of increasing awareness of pulses as a primary source of protein and other essential nutrients, as well as promoting expansion, discussion and cooperation at national, regional and global levels to increase awareness and understanding of the challenges faced by pulse growers (Global Pulse Confederation 2016). As more and more research is devoted to pulses and health, future work directed at the long term benefits of pulse consumption on diet quality and disease reduction coupled with efforts targeted toward increasing global consumption rates, particularly in Western society, would be critical to reinforce the role of pulses in a healthy diet.

## References

Al-Kanhal MA, Al-Mohizea IS, Al-Othaimeen AI et al (1998) Nutritional evaluation of some legume-based dishes consumed in Saudi Arabia. Int J Food Sci Nutr 49:193–197

Anderson JW, Smith BM, Washnock CS (1999) Cardiovascular and renal benefits of dry bean and soybean intake. Am J Clin Nutr 70:464s–474s

Aykroyd WL, Doughty J, Walker A (1964) Legumes in human nutrition. FAO Nutr. Studies, No. 19, Rome

Bekkering E (2015) Pulses in Canada. https://www150.statcan.gc.ca/n1/en/pub/96-325-x/2014001/article/14041-eng.pdf?st=RlcEyekB. Accessed 24 Nov 2018

Canadian Council on Social Development (2004) Visible minorities in Canada. Available at: http://www.ccsd.ca/resources/ProgressChildrenYouth/pdf/pccy_portrait.pdf Accessed 24 Nov 2018

Charlebois S (2017) New food guide will finally put consumers first. https://beta.theglobeandmail.com/opinion/new-food-guide-will-finally-put-consumers-first/article35751092/?ref=http://www.theglobeandmail.com& Accessed 24 Nov 2018

Coffmann CW, Garciaj VV (1977) Functional properties and amino acid content of a protein isolate from mung bean flour. Int J Food Sci Technol 12:473–484

Duyff RL, Mount JR, Jones JB (2011) Sodium reduction in canned beans after draining, rinsing. J Culinary Sci Technol 9:106–112

Eihusen J, Albrecht JA (2007) Dry bean intake of women ages 19–45. RURALS: Review of Undergraduate Research in Agricultural and. Life Sci 2:3

Faye S (2007) The pulse industry in Western Canada. http://www.assembly.ab.ca/lao/library/egov-docs/2007/alard/168746.pdf Accessed 24 Nov 2018

Food and Agricultural Organization (2016) Frequently asked questions. http://www.fao.org/pulses-2016/faq/en/ Accessed 24 Nov 2018

Fulgoni VL, Papanikolaou Y, Fulgoni SA et al (2006) Bean consumption by children is associated with better nutrient intake and lower body weights and waist circumferences. FASEB J 20:A621–A621

Global Pulse Confederation (2016) International year of pulses. http://iyp2016.org/ Accessed 24 Nov 2018

Health Canada (2008) Pulse symposium: investigating the nutrition and health attributes of beans, chickpeas, lentils, peas: clinical trial research projects funded by Canada's pulse industry. https://nutrition.uwo.ca/ibean/resources_healthbenefits_pulses.pdf. Accessed 28 Nov 2018

Health Canada (2010) Canada's food guide to healthy eating. http://www.hc-sc.gc.ca/fn-an/food-guide-aliment/using-utiliser/count-calcul-eng.php. Accessed 28 Nov 2018

Leterme P, Muñoz LC (2002) Factors influencing pulse consumption in Latin America. Br J Nutr 88(S3):251–254

Lucier G, Lin BH, Allshouse J et al (2000) Factors affecting dry bean consumption in the United States. Small 19:2–5

McCrory MA, Hamaker BR, Lovejoy JC et al (2010) Pulse consumption, satiety, and weight management. Adv Nutr 1:17–30

Mitchell DC, Lawrence FR, Hartman TJ et al (2009) Consumption of dry beans, peas, and lentils could improve diet quality in the US population. J Am Diet Assoc 109(5):909–913

Mudryj AN, Yu N, Hartman TJ et al (2012) Pulse consumption in Canadian adults influences nutrient intakes. Br J Nutr 108(S1):S27–S36

Mudryj AN, Yu N, Aukema HM (2014) Nutritional and health benefits of pulses. Appl Physiol Nutr Metab 39(11):1197–1204

Muzquiz M (1997) Spanish legumes and the Mediterranean diet. Grain Legumes 17:22–23

Ofuya ZM, Akhidue V (2005) The role of pulses in human nutrition: a review. J Appl Sci Environ Manag 9:99–104

Papanikolaou Y, Fulgoni VL III (2008) Bean consumption is associated with greater nutrient intake, reduced systolic blood pressure, lower body weight, and a smaller waist circumference in adults: results from the National Health and Nutrition Examination Survey 1999–2002. J Am Coll Nutr 27:569–576

Patterson CA, Maskus H, Dupasquier C (2009) Pulse crops for health: Pulse Canada. https://pdfs. semanticscholar.org/0180/ac583ede8f6c69cd0ef81eb3c05a46c88fe6.pdf. Accessed 28 Nov 2018

Pulse Canada (2017) Pulse industry. http://www.pulsecanada.com/producers-industry/. Accessed 28 Nov 2018

Saskatchewan Pulse Growers (2010) Overview of pulses. https://saskpulse.com/growing-pulses/. Accessed 28 Nov 2018

Schneider AV (2002) Overview of the market and consumption of pulses in Europe. Br J Nutr 88(S3):243–250

Statistics Canada (2007) Food statistics-2006. (Catalogue no. 21-020-X1E). Available at: http://www.statcan.gc.ca/pub/16-201-x/2009000/part-partie1-eng.htm

Tosh SM, Yada S (2010) Dietary fibres in pulse seeds and fractions: characterization, functional attributes, and applications. Food Res Int 43:450–460

United States Census Bureau (2017) Quick Facts. https://www.census.gov/quickfacts/fact/table/US/PST045217. Accessed 28 Nov 2018

U.S. Department of Agriculture (2017) Choose MyPlate. https://www.choosemyplate.gov/ Accessed 24 Nov 2018

U.S. Department of Health and Human Services and U.S. Department of Agriculture (n.d.) 2015–2020 dietary guidelines for Americans. 8th Edition. December 2015. https://health.gov/dietaryguidelines/2015/guidelines/. Accessed 28 Nov 2018

Winham D, Webb D, Barr A (2008) Beans and good health. Nutr Today 43:201–209

Zanovec M, O'Neil CE, Nicklas TA (2011) Comparison of nutrient density and nutrient-to-cost between cooked and canned beans. Food Nutr Sci 2:66

# Chapter 3
# Where Do Pulses Fit in Dietary Guidance Documents?

**Katherine Ford, Linda B. Bobroff, and Susan J. Whiting**

**Abstract** Pulses are plant-based sources of protein that offer many nutritional health benefits including fiber, vitamins, minerals, and bioactive compounds. This chapter presents the touted health benefits of pulses and the evidence behind these claims based on disease or condition affected. We also discuss dietary guidance documents from high-, middle-, and low-income countries, providing three examples of each, to show how pulses are included (or excluded) in promoting healthful dietary patterns. National and international associations and their use (or not) of pulses in dietary guidance are highlighted. A focus is placed on the inclusion of pulses (legumes) in American dietary guidelines.

**Keywords** Pulses · Legume · Dietary guidance · Food guide · Low-income countries · MyPlate · Dietary guidelines · Middle-income countries · Dietary recommendations

## 3.1 Introduction

Dietary guidance provides a means of promoting healthful diets to improve nutritional status and reduce risk of disease, especially chronic disease. Dietary guidance comes in a variety of forms. Many countries issue a food guide, which includes a pictorial of foods commonly consumed displayed in a way that encourages more healthy food choices compared to less healthy choices (FAO 2016). For example, in the United States, the federal government issued a food guide called MyPlate that promotes greater consumption of plant-based foods, among other nutrition

K. Ford · S. J. Whiting
College of Pharmacy and Nutrition, University of Saskatchewan, Saskatoon, SK, Canada
e-mail: katherine.ford@usask.ca; susan.whiting@usask.ca

L. B. Bobroff (✉)
Department of Family, Youth, and Community Sciences, University of Florida, Gainesville, FL, USA
e-mail: bobroff@ufl.edu

© Springer Nature Switzerland AG 2019
W. J. Dahl (ed.), *Health Benefits of Pulses*,
https://doi.org/10.1007/978-3-030-12763-3_3

messages designed to improve eating patterns, promote optimal health, and reduce disease risk (USDA n.d.). A country may also set dietary guidelines that focus on a series of statements related to healthy eating (FAO 2016). For example, Sweden uses three messages focused on what to consume more of, less of, and food items to switch to (such as whole grains, healthier fat, and low-fat dairy). Finally, national or international health-related societies are now setting guidelines related to prevention and treatment of particular diseases, with some messages including diet or nutrition. In the United States, the American Heart Association provides specific diet and lifestyle recommendations related to heart disease (AHA n.d.).

Pulses are foods that have been eaten worldwide for thousands of years (Mudryj et al. 2014). Pulses are a part of the Leguminosae (legume) family and include dried beans (e.g., black beans, chickpeas or garbanzo beans, kidney beans, and lima beans), dried peas, and lentils (Bareja 2016). Conversely, fresh beans and peas, soybeans, peanuts, and soy nuts are not considered pulses, but are still classified as a part of the legume family. The high fat content of soybeans, soy nuts, and peanuts is the main difference between these legumes and above-mentioned pulses, as the latter's fat content is negligible. Fresh beans and peas are considered vegetables rather than pulses because they are harvested in their green state. Pulses are harvested in their dried grain state, and for this reason are sometimes called "grain legumes" (Bareja 2016).

Pulses are touted as a plant-based source of protein, but they offer other nutritional benefits including fiber, vitamins, minerals, and bioactive compounds. There are other benefits to consuming a diet rich in plant-based proteins. Ranganathan et al. (2016) suggest that a shift away from animal-based proteins (beef, specifically) to plant-based proteins will aid in creating a sustainable food environment into the future. Additionally, pulses play an important agricultural role as they require little to no nitrogen fertilizer and decrease the carbon footprint emitted by other crops, when used in a rotating sequence (Mudryj et al. 2014; Burgess et al. 2012; Gan et al. 2011; Harrison 2011; Foyer et al. 2016). Thus, there are both nutritional and environmental advantages of promoting pulses as a food crop.

In 2016, the Food and Agriculture Organization of the United Nations declared 2016 to be "The Year of the Pulse." It would seem reasonable for pulses to be included in food guidance as a way to encourage the consumption of this inexpensive yet environmentally friendly and healthful food. Therefore, we examined dietary guidance in the United States as well as in selected countries of differing socioeconomic status to determine the prominence of pulse foods in each system, and whether there is specific pulse food messaging in each food guide.

## 3.2 Health Benefits of Pulses

Research has indicated that adding pulses to the diet improves many aspects of human health. Table 3.1 summarizes research focused on the nutritional and health benefits of pulses. Foremost, being a consumer of pulses, defined as having at least

**Table 3.1**  Nutritional and health benefits of pulses

| Benefit type | Disease or condition affected | Nature of evidence |
|---|---|---|
| Improvement in nutrient intake | Reduction in dietary inadequacy of thiamin, vitamin B6, folate, iron, magnesium, phosphorus, and zinc | Canadian adults in national survey |
| | Improvement in dietary intake of fiber, protein, folate, zinc, iron, and magnesium | American adults in national survey data |
| Reduction in chronic disease risk | Colorectal cancer: negative association with fiber intake | Comprehensive review by WCRF/AICR |
| | Cardiovascular disease (CVD); inverse relationship with pulse intake | National survey follow-up data |
| | Anti-hypertensive effect: blood pressure reduction | Meta-analysis of human trials |
| | Type 2 diabetes: improvement in glucose tolerance and insulin sensitivity | Meta-analysis of human trials |
| Weight management | Obesity prevention: increased satiety | Randomized trials |
| | Obesity treatment: reduction in waist circumference | Randomized trials |
| HIV | Improvement in immune function: phagocytosis of macrophages | Analysis of lectin properties of pulses |
| Aging | Increased longevity: extended life expectancy | Prospective cohort studies |
| Stress | Reduced anxiety | Epidemiology |

Adapted from: Mudryj et al. 2014

one serving of pulses daily, improves intake of macronutrients such as protein and fiber, and micronutrients, including iron, zinc, folate, and magnesium. Notably, fiber, zinc, and magnesium are nutrients that are low in the diets of Americans (Fulgoni et al. 2011) and of Canadians (Mudryj et al. 2016) who do not consume pulses. Folate is a nutrient of concern for women of child-bearing age due to its role in reducing risk of neural tube defects in infants; inadequate folate intake remains a problem in countries lacking folic acid fortification, such as the United Kingdom (Khoshnood et al. 2015).

In terms of reducing risk of chronic disease, Table 3.1 shows that pulse consumption is associated with reduction in risk of colorectal cancer, cardiovascular disease (CVD), hypertension, and type 2 diabetes. Randomized controlled trials have identified strong cause and effect relationships between increased pulse consumption and a reduction in the severity of hypertension and diabetes (Mudryj et al. 2014). Pulses are also being studied for contribution to weight management, possibly due to the satiety effect of the high fiber/high protein content of pulse foods. As obesity is a risk factor for many chronic diseases (WHO 2017) this is an important health benefit of consuming a diet rich in pulses. Evidence is emerging of positive effects of pulse intake in areas other than chronic disease such as HIV susceptibility (enhanced immune function), stress reduction, and longevity (Mudryj et al. 2014).

## 3.3   Dietary Guidance: International

Given the growing body of evidence that pulses can play a role in improving the health of populations by reducing chronic disease, among other health benefits, it is important that countries promote pulse intake in their national dietary guidelines. Across countries, dietary guidance by the federal government often includes published dietary guidelines that include a food guide. The Food and Agriculture Organization of the United Nations (FAO) provides a website where one may search for and read dietary guidance documents from countries in all regions of the world (FAO 2016). Table 3.2 highlights some examples of food guides from countries that are high income countries (HIC), middle income countries (MIC), and low-income countries (LIC) (World Bank n.d.). The food guide from the United States, a HIC, is shown in Table 3.3. Almost all countries, despite income differences, had pulses or legumes in their food guides.

The MyPlate icon, representing the United States food guide does not show pulses, or any food, as part of its plate image. In the text of the Dietary Guidelines for Americans, it is noted that legumes can be classified as both a protein and a vegetable (USDA n.d.). This duality is both a plus and a minus – it acknowledges that pulses are good sources of protein and also sources of vitamins, minerals, and fiber that are found in many vegetables. However, it makes the classification and inclusion of pulses difficult in dietary guidelines. Therefore, pulses are likely to be omitted in an attempt to simplify dietary information.

Another issue with pulses is the notion that they are a "poor person's meat" (Iriti and Varoni 2017). This attitude is observed in western countries (Iriti and Varoni 2017) as well as in low income countries such as Ethiopia (Kabata et al. 2017). This perception stigmatizes pulses and makes them less appealing to the rising low-middle classes where meat may be viewed as a sign of economic success. While many authors are now writing about the important role that plant-based proteins play in human health and in environmental sustainability (Foyer et al. 2016), without overcoming the stigma of pulses as a poor person's meat, it will be difficult to encourage increased consumption in certain populations. In Table 3.2, it can be seen that the food guide from Benin and the food guide from Canada classify pulses as meat 'alternatives.' The term 'alternative' may imply that pulses should only be consumed when meat products are unavailable. Denoting pulses as 'alternatives' may add to the stigma already associated with these foods. In fact, the Benin food guide states: "When there is no meat, fish or eggs… you can replace them with pulses, peanuts, soybeans, soya, cheese or peas" (FAO 2016). In order to increase consumption of pulses, they must be promoted as healthful foods, equal in stature to other healthful food sources of protein, by being included pictorially in food guides, wherever foods are included (e.g., not on the MyPlate icon).

**Table 3.2** Examples of dietary food guides worldwide

| Ranking[a] | Country | Dietary guideline | Year | How pulses[b] are displayed in food guide[c] |
|---|---|---|---|---|
| *High income countries* | | | | |
| | Canada | Canada's food guide (4 food groups) | 2007 | Beans and lentils shown in group called Meat and Alternatives; relevant dietary message is "Have meat alternatives such as beans, lentils and tofu often" |
| | Japan | Spinning top (5 food groups) | 2010 | Pulses are not shown. Protein group is labeled fish and meat dishes. Relevant dietary message is: "Combine vegetables, fruits, milk products, beans and fish in your diet" |
| | Netherlands | Wheel of 5 (5 food groups) | 2015 | Pulses not found in food groups; relevant dietary message is "Eat legumes weekly" |
| *Middle income countries* | | | | |
| | China | Food guide pagoda (4 food groups) | 2016 | Pulses not shown. Relevant dietary message is: "A daily diet should include…soybeans and nuts" |
| | India | Food pyramid (4 food groups) | 2011 | Cereals and legumes/beans are at the base of the pyramid. "Cereals, millets and pulses are major sources of most nutrients" |
| | South Africa | Interlocking circles (6 food groups) | 2012 | Dry beans, split peas, lentils and soya are one food group. Relevant dietary message is: "Eat dry beans, split peas, lentils and soya regularly" |
| *Low income countries* | | | | |
| | Benin | Traditional African house (5 food groups) | 2015 | Cereals/tubers; plant/animal-protein foods are the foods at the base. Relevant dietary message: "When there is no meat, fish or eggs… you can replace them with pulses, peanuts, soybeans, soya, cheese or peas" |
| | Namibia | Food and nutrition guidelines (4 food groups) | 2000 | Dried beans and peas are found with meat and fish. Relevant dietary message: "Eat beans or meat regularly" |
| | Sierra Leone | Food-based dietary guidelines for healthy eating | 2016 | One of the 6 food groups is called: "beans, peas, and lentils". Relevant dietary message: "Eat either beans, peas and lentils every day" |

[a]World Bank ranking of countries: https://blogs.worldbank.org/opendata/lics-lmics-umics-and-hics-classifying-economies-analytical-purposes
[b]Use of "pulse" also considers related terms such as legumes
[c]Food guide information from: http://www.fao.org/nutrition/education/food-dietary-guidelines/regions/

**Table 3.3** Where pulses (legumes) fit in American Dietary Guidelines

| Major dietary guidance for Americans | Where pulses fit | Organization website |
|---|---|---|
| MyPlate | Pulses are a component of both the protein and vegetable categories of MyPlate; in recognition of this duality there is a subsection in the document called "Beans and peas are unique foods" | ChooseMyPlate.gov |
| Dietary Approaches to Stop Hypertension (DASH) diet | Legumes are a category of food that is recommended to be consumed on a weekly basis | nhlbi.nih.gov |
| American Heart Association | Suggest "Nuts and Legumes" as part of an overall healthy eating pattern | heart.org |
| American Diabetes Association | Carbohydrate intake from legumes is recommended over other sources of carbohydrates | diabetes.org |
| American Cancer Society | Emphasizes plant foods but does not specifically mention pulses or legumes | cancer.org |
| 2015–2020 Dietary Guidelines for Americans | Legumes are mentioned as vegetable and protein foods that are a part of a healthy eating pattern | health.gov |

## 3.4 Dietary Guidance in the United States: Government and Non-governmental Organizations

Given the impetus to promote plant sources of protein (Ranganathan et al. 2016), one would expect some degree of prominence given to pulse foods in dietary guidance. This section examines dietary recommendations for risk reduction related to chronic disease in the United States.

Dietary guidance in the United States was first released in the form of a food guide in 1916. Since that time, the original food guide has been altered eight times and is now called MyPlate. When the food guide was originally issued, the focus was on food groups and household measures. In the 1940s, the guide evolved to be more complex and highlighted seven groups that aimed at individuals attaining nutritional adequacy. More than a decade later, the food guide was simplified from seven food groups to four, but it remained focused on obtaining nutritional adequacy. In 1979, a new food guide was released with the same four food groups and an additional group highlighting that intake of fats, sugars, and alcohol should be moderated. Moderation as well as nutrient adequacy has been a consistent focus of food guides in the US since the 1980s. In 1992, the Food Guide Pyramid was introduced, and in 2005, it was dramatically changed to MyPyramid. In 2011, a plate showing the names of the five main food groups (fruits, vegetables, protein, grains, dairy) became the latest USDA food guide (USDA n.d.). The Dietary Guidelines for Americans (DGA), from the US Department of Agriculture and the US Department of Health and Human Services are issued approximately every 5 years and are based on current scientific knowledge (DHHS n.d.). They aim to assist Americans in making healthy food and beverage choices to promote health and reduce disease risk. The 2015–2020 DGA suggest that legumes are an important component of a healthy eating pattern and can be classified as both vegetable and protein foods. The guidelines have a subsection called *About Legumes (Beans and Peas)* that explains what foods are considered legumes, the health benefits of legumes, why they are classified as both vegetables and proteins, and why green peas and beans are not classified as legumes, a common misconception (DHHS n.d.). Additional practical information about incorporating pulses (legumes) into the diet is found on the MyPlate website, ChooseMyPlate.gov.

The Dietary Approaches to Stop Hypertension (DASH) diet was originally designed to have blood pressure lowering effects, but has since claimed to also have positive effects on weight loss and general health. DASH is supported by the National Heart, Lung, and Blood Institute of the National Institutes of Health. This dietary approach focuses on eating whole foods with an emphasis on fruits and vegetables, low-fat and non-fat dairy, whole grains, lean meats, fish and poultry, and nuts, beans, and seeds. Nuts, seeds, and legumes are a specific category of food in the DASH diet, but their recommended consumption is based on weekly intake whereas the other food groups are recommended for daily intake (NHLBI 2015).

Other dietary guidance is issued in the United States as part of the work of medically-based societies and associations. We searched guidelines from those societies/associations related to the chronic diseases identified in Table 3.1. As seen in Table 3.3, we identified three dietary guidance documents issued by medically-based societies and associations including the American Heart Association, the American Diabetes Association, and the American Cancer Society.

Although the DASH diet has been shown to aid in lowering cholesterol, the American Heart Association has released their own set of dietary guidelines (and lifestyle recommendations) to promote heart health (AHA n.d.). Nuts and legumes are included in the healthy eating pattern suggested by the AHA. A subsection of these guidelines describes specific details about the benefits of beans and legumes and suggests simple ways of adding them into the diet (AHA n.d.). Overall, the dietary guidelines released by the AHA are quite similar to those of the DASH diet and promote a shift towards lean animal proteins and plant-based proteins (AHA n.d.).

The American Diabetes Association releases nutrition therapy recommendations that focus on achieving optimal glycemic control and reduced risk for cardiovascular disease for persons with diabetes. The recommendations are extensive and cover many aspects of nutrition therapy. Of note, the recommendations suggest that "Carbohydrate intake from vegetables, fruits, whole grains, legumes, and dairy products should be advised over intake from other carbohydrate sources…" (American Diabetes Association 2015).

The American Cancer Society has issued Nutrition and Physical Activity Guidelines that are in line with the previously discussed guidelines set by the American Heart Association and the American Diabetes Association. Although these guidelines emphasize the inclusion of plant-based foods in a healthy diet, the guidelines do not specifically mention pulses or legumes (Kushi et al. 2012).

# References

American Diabetes Association (2015) Foundations of care: education, nutrition, physical activity, smoking cessation, psychosocial care, and immunization. Diabetes Care 38(Suppl 1):S20–S30

American Heart Association (AHA) (n.d.) The American Heart Association's diet and lifestyle recommendations. http://www.heart.org/HEARTORG/HealthyLiving/Diet-and-Lifestyle-Recommendations_UCM_305855_Article.jsp#.Wd1NZDjrtv4. Accessed 4 Aug 2017

Bareja BG (2016) List of pulses or grain legumes and their various names. http://www.cropsreview.com/grain-legumes.html. Accessed 1 Aug 2017

Burgess MH, Miller PR, Jones CA (2012) Pulse crops improve energy intensity and productivity of cereal production in Montana, U.S.A. J Sustain Agric 36:699–718

Department of Human Health Services (DHHS) (n.d.) Dietary guidelines for Americans. https://www.hhs.gov/fitness/eat-healthy/dietary-guidelines-for-americans/index.html

Food and Agriculture Organization (2016) Food-based dietary guidelines. http://www.fao.org/nutrition/education/food-dietary-guidelines/regions/. Accessed 31 Jul 2017

Foyer CH, Lam HM, Nguyen HT et al (2016) Neglecting legumes has compromised human health and sustainable food production. Nat Plants 2:16112

Fulgoni VL, Keast DR, Bailey RL et al (2011) Foods, fortificants, and supplements: where do Americans get their nutrients? J Nutr 141:1847–1854

Gan Y, Liang C, Wang X et al (2011) Lowering carbon footprint of durum wheat by diversifying cropping systems. Field Crops Res 122:199–206

Harrison M (2011) Pulse crops may reduce energy use and increase yields for farmers. http://www.physorg.com/news/2011-05-pulse-crops-energy-yields-farmers.html. Accessed 31 Jul 2017

Iriti M, Varoni EM (2017) Pulses, healthy, and sustainable food sources for feeding the planet. Int J Mol Sci 18:255–260

Kabata A, Henry C, Moges D et al (2017) Determinants and constraints of pulse production and consumption among farming households of Ethiopia. J Food Res 6:41–49

Khoshnood B, Loane M, de Walle H et al (2015) Long term trends in prevalence of neural tube defects in Europe: population based study. BMJ 351:h5949

Kushi LH, Doyle C, McCullough M et al (2012) American Cancer Society guidelines on nutrition and physical activity for cancer prevention: reducing the risk of cancer with healthy food choices and physical activity. CA Cancer J Clin 62:30–67

Mudryj AN, Yu N, Hartman TJ, Mitchell DC et al (2012) Pulse consumption in Canadian adults influences nutrient intakes. BJN 108:S27–S36

Mudryj AN, Yu N, Aukema HM (2014) Nutritional and health benefits of pulses. Appl Physiol Nutr Metab 39:1197–1204

Mudryj AN, Aukema HM, Fieldhouse P et al (2016) Nutrient and food group intakes of Manitoba children and youth: a population-based analysis by pulse and soy consumption status. Can J Diet Pract Res 77:189–194

National Heart, Lung, and Blood Institute (NHLBI) (2015) Description of the DASH eating plan. https://www.nhlbi.nih.gov/health/health-topics/topics/dash. Accessed 2 Nov 2017

Ranganathan J, Vennard D, Waite R et al (2016) Shifting diets for a sustainable food future, Working Paper, Installment 11 of "Creating a Sustainable Food Future". World Resources Institute, Washington, DC. http://www.wri.org/sites/default/files/Shifting_Diets_for_a_Sustainable_Food_Future_0.pdf. Accessed 2 Nov 2017

U.S. Department of Agriculture (n.d.-a) Beans and peas are unique foods. https://www.choosemyplate.gov/vegetables-beans-and-peas. Accessed 2 Aug 2017

U.S. Department of Agriculture (n.d.-b) A brief history of USDA food guides. https://choosemyplate-prod.azureedge.net/sites/default/files/printablematerials/ABriefHistoryOfUSDAFoodGuides.pdf. Accessed 2 Aug 2017

World Bank (n.d.) New country classifications by income level: 2018–2019. https://blogs.worldbank.org/opendata/new-country-classifications-income-level-2018-2019

World Health Organization (2017) Global Health Observatory (GHO) data: obesity 2008. http://www.who.int/gho/ncd/risk_factors/obesity_text/en/. Accessed 31 Jul 2017

# Chapter 4
# Pulses and Mineral Bioavailability in Low Income Countries

Susan J. Whiting, Getenesh Berhanu, Hiwot Abebe Haileslassie, and Carol J. Henry

**Abstract** Pulse crops are important sources of nutrients in low income countries (LIC). Not only do they provide good sources of proteins when mixed with cereals, but they also contain good to very good sources of key minerals such as iron, zinc and calcium. These minerals are important for growth and development of children as well as women's health. Pulses, however, contain phytate and polyphenols, and these can bind to divalent minerals and prevent absorption, thus limiting bioavailability. Home processing methods of soaking, germination and fermentation can reduce the effects of phytate and polyphenols.

**Keywords** Pulses · Legume · Micronutrient · Bioavailability · Antinutrients · Phytate · Biofortification · Calcium · Iron · Zinc

## 4.1 Introduction

Micronutrient deficiency, also known as "hidden hunger," is a major public health problem in most developing countries, with iron, calcium and zinc among the micronutrients of greatest concern. As pulses improve both macro- and micro-nutrient status, it is of interest to examine the contribution pulses may make to mineral nutrition. However, research has shown that there are many anti-nutrients in pulse foods, and that removal of these compounds is needed or else the bioavailability of minerals is low. Bioavailability is the term used to describe "the proportion of a dietary nutrient that is absorbed and utilized through normal metabolic pathways" (Hurrell 2002, p. 5), and acknowledges that not just the quantity of a nutrients but their retention that is critical for nutrient status. In this chapter, "bioavailability" is being more narrowly defined as "the amount of ingested nutrient that is potentially available for absorption, is dependent only on digestion and

S. J. Whiting (✉) · G. Berhanu · H. A. Haileslassie · C. J. Henry
College of Pharmacy and Nutrition, University of Saskatchewan, Saskatoon, SK, Canada
e-mail: susan.whiting@usask.ca; cj.henry@usask.ca

© Springer Nature Switzerland AG 2019
W. J. Dahl (ed.), *Health Benefits of Pulses*,
https://doi.org/10.1007/978-3-030-12763-3_4

release from food matrix" (Etcheverry et al. 2002, p. 1). This is due to the anti-nutrient factors in pulses, i.e. phytate and polyphenols, acting solely in the gastro-intestinal tract.

Anti-nutrients that are present in significant amounts in pulses include proteinase inhibitors (e.g. trypsin inhibitors), oxalate, lectins, raffinose oligosaccharides, saponins, amylase inhibitor, polyphenols and phytate (Costa et al. 2006). Most of the anti-nutrients that affect protein digestibility are heat sensitive, thus cooking alone was found to be useful in improving protein digestibility in pulse-based diets (Nergiz and Gökgöz 2007). On the other hand, phytic acid and polyphenols (including tannins) have the capacity to withstand heat, and thus are categorized as heat stable anti-nutrients. They are among the anti-nutrients of greatest concern with regards to mineral bioavailability. They form complexes with minerals, rendering them less available or unavailable for absorption. Thus, the purpose of this chapter is to describe how pulses may contribute to key micromineral intakes provided processing or other strategies to reduce anti-nutrients are implemented.

## 4.2   Mineral Content of Pulses

In countries where protein is difficult to obtain in the diet, pulse-cereal blends are often used to get sources of good quality protein. Indeed, in developing countries, pulses contribute to energy intake to a great extent, second only to cereals (Siddiq and Uebersax 2012). Pulses also contribute to the overall intake of many minerals. The chemical composition of pulses, however, varies based on climatic conditions, nutrient content and pH of soil, location, and genotype (Ray et al. 2014). This is true not only for nutrient composition, but to anti-nutrient composition as well (Petry et al. 2010).

The focus for human nutrition is in key minerals that are low in diets of low-income countries (LIC) (Gibson et al. 2006) and high-income countries (HIC) (Fulgoni et al. 2011), namely calcium, iron and zinc, as these greatly affect health and wellbeing of women and children worldwide. Further, these minerals are cations adversely affected by phytate and polyphenols. Table 4.1 provides food composition data showing levels of these key minerals (iron, zinc and calcium) in commonly consumed pulses. By consuming just one serving a day of pulse (100 g cooked weight), one can obtain 5% of Dietary Value (DV) for calcium, 10–15% of DV for iron, and close to 10% of DV for zinc. However, bioavailability would be low unless steps were taken to reduce phytate and tannin levels. This is a great concern in most developing countries that largely depend on plant-based staple diets (Hotz and Gibson 2007). For example, Zimmermann et al. (2005) showed that in children, despite a seemingly high iron intake, absorption was only 2% compared to 10% from a mixed animal and plant-based diet (Zimmermann et al. 2005).

**Table 4.1** Nutrient composition of whole, dried, boiled pulses in terms of 100 g edible portion and percentage of United States Dietary Value (DV) (Ethiopia Health and Nutrition Research Institute (EHNRI) 1997), Food Composition Table for use in Ethiopia. Part III, USDA 2017, Umeta et al. 2005)

| Pulses | Energy | Calcium | Iron | Zinc |
|---|---|---|---|---|
| | kcal | Mg | | |
| 10% DV[a] | 200 | 130 | 1.8 | 1.5 |
| Broad bean | 150 | 54 | 2.9 | 1.0 |
| Haricot bean | 170 | 65 | 3.3 | 1.0 |
| Chickpea | 181 | 96 | 2.2 | 1.5 |
| Lentil | 153 | 25 | 2.1 | 1.3 |
| Pea | 158 | 47 | 1.9 | 1.0 |

[a]DV values found at Food and Drug Administration (FDA) Available at: https://www.fda.gov:80/FDAgov/Food/GuidanceRegulation/GuidanceDocumentsRegulatoryInformation/LabelingNutrition/ucm064928.htm

## 4.3 Phytate and Pulses

The molecule myo-inositol hexakisphosphate (IP6) is commonly called phytate, having the chemical formula $C_6H_{18}O_{24}P_6$ (Oatway et al. 2001). "Phytate" is the salt form, whereas when it is in the acid form, the molecule is termed "phytic acid" (Ali et al. 2010). Phytate is the main storage unit for phosphate and inositol in plants and is essential for seed germination and plant growth. In the case of pulses, phytate accumulates in the cotyledon (Bohn et al. 2008). Phytate concentration in plants can vary based on the location, year of cultivation, genotype, rain or drought, high temperature and pathogens (Bohn et al. 2008).

The impact of phytate on mineral bioavailability is dose dependent (Hurrell and Egli 2010), thus reduction of phytate in food will help to increase bioavailability. The negatively charged phosphate groups in phytate gives it the capacity to chelate divalent cations such as calcium, magnesium, zinc, and iron (Bohn et al. 2008). The complex formed between phytate and minerals has low solubility at the pH of the intestine and as these minerals are no longer in an ionic form, carrier proteins located on the intestinal cell membrane cannot bind and transport them (Lopez et al. 2002). It is necessary to hydrolyse the complex to be able to utilize the mineral bound with the phytate, but this needs the enzyme phytase, which sequentially removes phosphate groups. Phytate (Ip6) needs to be degraded to inositol phosphate lower than IP-3 (three remaining phosphate groups) in order to increase mineral absorption (Sandberg 2002). Phytase can be obtained from different sources that include plants, microbes, small intestinal mucosa and gut microbial flora (Kumar et al. 2010). However, it is not present in the human gut in significant amounts. Unless broken down, the insoluble phytate-mineral complex is excreted via the stool (Lönnerdal 2000).

Table 4.2 provides phytate levels for some common pulses. As previously described, there is a large variation in content due to multiple reasons. Values shown in Table 4.2 vary between fourfold and sixfold for the same variety, while kidney beans have almost double the level as the other pulses listed. Phytate reduces absorp-

**Table 4.2** Phytate content in pulse crops and other legumes by dry weight (DW) (Gupta et al. 2015)

| Pulses | Phytic acid |
|---|---|
| | g/100 (DW) |
| Kidney beans | 0.61–2.38 |
| Chickpeas | 0.28–1.60 |
| Peas | 0.22–1.22 |
| Lentils | 0.27–1.51 |

**Table 4.3** Optimal phytate-to-mineral ratios (mol:mol) (Gibson et al. 2010)

| Mineral | Ratio |
|---|---|
| Phytate: iron | <1.0 |
| Phytate: zinc | <18 |
| Phytate: calcium | <0.17 |

tion of calcium, iron and zinc differentially. Molar ratios have been determined (Table 4.3). These show that zinc is most affected, followed by iron, with calcium being relatively unaffected unless a very large amount of phytate is present (Gibson 2011). Ways to reduce phytate contact are described below.

## 4.4 Polyphenols and Tannins

Polyphenols in plants are large molecules having diverse functions that are concentrated throughout the plant. There are 1000's of these molecules and they range from 1% to 25% total natural phenols dry mass (Manach et al. 2004) in foods such as cereals, legumes, vegetables, fruits, tea, coffee and wine, and impart an astringent taste to these foods. Plant phenols include simple phenols, coumarins, flavonoids, phenolic acids, stilbenes and tannins (Naczk and Shahidi 2004). Tannins, especially, are capable of binding divalent cations such as iron, rendering it less bioavailable (Sandberg 2002). Despite their anti-nutritive impacts, polyphenols are useful for plants as they have a role in defending against pathogens and pests. In addition, research is ongoing on beneficial properties of polyphenols to human health (Fraga et al. 2010).

Polyphenols are found in pulses, particularly in seed hulls, and also in higher quantities in colored varieties (Petry et al. 2010). In LIC pulses may be consumed without dehulling, and the impact on mineral absorption may be more severe than in HIC countries where other, more bioavailable sources of iron, zinc and calcium may be ingested, for example as animal source foods. Thus, it is important to determine how polyphenols in pulses affect mineral bioavailability. To answer this question, Petry et al. (2010) performed a series of studies using beans with varying amounts of polyphenols. As shown in Fig. 4.1, when 20 mg of polyphenols derived from bean hulls were given to iron deficient subjects along with stable isotopes of

**Fig. 4.1**  Iron absorption in iron-deficient women given different doses of polyphenols (PP) from bean hulls. At 20 mg PP, there was no change in iron absorption; at 50 mg and 200 mg PP, iron absorption was reduced to 84% and 55% of normal, respectively (Petry et al. 2010)

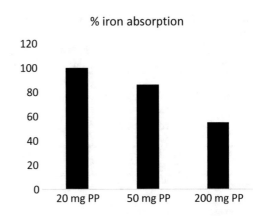

% iron absorption

iron, iron absorption remained normal; however, at 50 mg PP and 200 mg PP, iron absorption fell to 84% and 55% of normal, respectively. In the same study, other experiments showed a decline in iron absorption with phytate, in a manner that indicated there was no additive effect seen with phytate and polyphenols.

## 4.5   Processing to Improve Bioavailability of Minerals from Pulses

In LIC where pulse intakes are critical to maintain proper nutrition, household food preparation and processing methods such as germination, fermentation and soaking can be used to reduce phytate (Gupta et al. 2015). Some of these may also reduce polyphenol effects, and in particular, dehulling as a first stage in pulse processing reduces polyphenol content (Petry et al. 2010).

Soaking of pulse crops in water reduces phytate concentration due to passive diffusion of phytate. Soaking also facilitates the activation of phytase, the extent of phytate removal through soaking depends on pH, temperature and duration of soaking (Hotz and Gibson 2007). Table 4.4 shows a number of studies where soaking followed by cooking reduced phytate, polyphenol and tannin concentrations in various pulses (Haileslassie et al. 2016). A long soaking time was not necessarily best. Soaking for 12 hours produced 50–80% reduction in these anti-nutrients.

Germination is the process of soaking of pulse seeds in water until they sprout. Germination activates endogenous phytases (Hotz and Gibson 2007). Reduction of phytate due to germination depends variety, pH, moisture content, temperature and solubility of phytate. Germination has the advantage of improving consistency of porridge mixtures made for young children as complementary foods. Porridge prepared from mixture of germinated and ungerminated flour has semi-liquid consistency which is suitable for young child feeding and has higher energy and nutrient density (Hotz and Gibson 2007). A review of germination studies shows reduction in phytate, polyphenols and tannins with 24 or 48 hours of germination, with no clear picture as to which time is better.

**Table 4.4** Effect of soaking and cooking on the anti-nutrient content of beans (Haileslassie et al. 2016)

| Study (first author) | Type of bean, country | Soaking time | Phytate reduction | Tannin reduction | Polyphenols reduction |
|---|---|---|---|---|---|
| | | hours | % | | |
| Khattab | Red kidney bean, Canada | 4 | 58 | | |
| Rehman | Red kidney bean, Pakistan | 4 | 24 | 24–27 | – |
| Yasmin | Red kidney bean, Pakistan | 9 | n.s.[a] | 82 | 61 |
| Nergiz | White kidney bean, Turkey | 12 | 57–58 | 81–82 | 73–78 |
| Shimelis | Kidney bean, Ethiopia | 12 | 61–65 | 58–70 | – |
| Greiner | Kidney beans, Brazil | 15 | 16–24 | – | – |
| Xu | Black bean, U.S.A. | 16 | – | – | 26–77 |
| El Maki | White bean, Egypt | 24 | 2–9 | – | 1–16 |
| Chimmad | Black bean, India | 24 | 22 | 39 | 59 |
| El Maki | White bean, Egypt | 36 | 4–16 | – | 13–23 |
| | | 48 | 3–12 | – | 6–22 |

Soaking occurred as 1:3–1:5 seed:water ratio

–, not reported

[a]*n.s.* not significant effect

Fermentation reduces phytate through the action of microbial phytase enzymes. Over 90% of phyate can be removed during fermentation in cereals and pulse crops (Hotz and Gibson 2007). In addition, fermentation improves protein digestibility thus making this an appropriate complementary food (Egli et al. 2002). During fermentation citric and lactic acids are produced which help to enhance bioavailability of iron and zinc.

Soaking, germination and fermentation require time and water, which often rural women in LIC do not have in abundance. However, we found that rural women in Ethiopia reported that processing of pulse crops through soaking and germination prior to cooking, reduced cooking time and therefore need for firewood (Henry et al. 2016). Another consideration is nutrient loss with these methods, as vitamins and minerals may leach into the water which is subsequently thrown out. Haileslassie et al. (2016) noted that the effect of soaking and germination on iron and zinc content was mixed in the studies reviewed; some losses were reported, but effects were not consistent. In addition, storage conditions may reduce the phytate content of intact legumes due to the intrinsic phytase enzyme activity. The decrease in InsP6 of 7% in beans has been reported after storage at 41 °C and 75% humidity for 3 months when compared to storage at room temperature (Gibson et al. 2018).

## 4.6   Biofortification

As intake of minerals from plant-based foods may be limiting, biofortification is the development of crop varieties rich in vitamin and mineral content. There are proven agricultural strategies to improve the nutrient contents of plants which include the use of fertilizer, plant breeding, and genetic engineering (Welch and Graham 2004). There is progress in breeding for better micronutrient levels, for example iron-biofortified beans. A feeding trial, conducted over 4.5 months using iron-biofortified bean, improved the iron status of Rwandan women (Haas et al. 2016). The next challenging steps in biofortification are demonstrating its effectiveness and scaling up (Ruel and Alderman 2013). In terms of improving mineral bioavailability, Petry et al. (2010) argue that biofortified crops containing more of these key mineral elements may be more effective at reducing mineral deficiencies that breeding out phytate and/or polyphenols.

A further consideration is that minerals may compete with each other at the site of absorption, thus coming in the way of their bioavailability. It has been previously reported that exogenous both iron and calcium at the therapeutic levels significantly reduced the bioavailability of zinc. Thus zinc supplementation should be considered along with that of iron and calcium (Platel and Srinivasan 2016).

## 4.7   Techniques for Measurement of Mineral Bioavailability

Many methods and models are used to determine the bioavailability of minerals, and may involve one or more of algorithms, in vitro studies and in vivo studies. Those that are in vivo use meals labelled with either a radioisotope or staple isotope nutrient; when provided to study participants, there are follow-up biological collections (blood, stool, and/or urine) to assess the uptake of the nutrient of interest. Indirect non-isotopic methods such as chemical balance, changes in hemoglobin and serum ferritin and zinc have also been used to assess bioavailability in human studies. In vivo studies, however, are expensive and ethical issues are of great concern. Animal models such as rat pups have been used for zinc bioavailability due to their lower phytase compared to adult rats; however, their immature gut limits their full utilization (Hotz 2005). For iron bioavailability, rat models are not as useful as in case of zinc as rodents are able to synthesise ascorbic acid, unlike humans. In vitro methods include solubility, dialyzability gastrointestinal model and Caco-2 cells. Solubility of iron at pH simulating gastrointestinal digestion suffers from replicating the physiological conditions of intestine and results were not well correlated with human studies (Pynaert et al. 2006). Dialyzability, measure of dialyzable mineral, is a better predictor of bioavailability than solubility. However, it has a low reproducibility (Fairweather-Tait et al. 2007) and does not measure uptake.

As described above, measurement of mineral bioavailability can be done in vivo in humans using stable isotope techniques (Petry et al. 2010), however, this is expensive. There are in vivo or in situ animal models, yet determining bioavailability with direct application to the human situation is difficult. Caco-2 cells, a human colon carcinoma cell line, differentiate into polarized, monolayer cells that exhibit features of intestinal cells when they are cultured. They are used as a cost effective, rapid in vitro tool for determining iron or zinc bioavailability (García-Nebot et al. 2013). Dietary factors that are known to affect iron absorption in human studies showed similar effects on iron uptake when compared to studies that utilized Caco-2 cells. Yun et al. (2004) reported that the absorption ratio increased with an increase in ascorbic acid whereas it decreased with tannic acid. The inhibitory effect of phytic acid on iron absorption has been demonstrated using Caco-2 cells (Glahn et al. 2002). Iron bioavailability of lentil measured using caco-2 cell showed similar result in an in vivo study (Tako et al. 2011). To our knowledge no studies of zinc availability from pulses has been demonstrated using this cell line, but future studies may focus on this. Overall this method has the potential to test many different combinations of food factors to determine bioavailability of iron or zinc. Further, bioavailability of minerals could be determined by using in vitro method where gastrointestinal digestion simulated. By using this in vitro method, it has been shown that allium spices onion and garlic, which are rich in sulfur-containing compounds, enhanced bioavailability of iron and zinc in pulses (Platel and Srinivasan 2016) (Table 4.5).

**Table 4.5** Effect of germination (25–30 °C) on the anti-nutrient content of uncooked or cooked beans (Haileslassie et al. 2016)

| Source | Types of bean, country | Cooking | Germi-nation | Phytate reduction | Tannin reduction | Polyphenols reduction |
|---|---|---|---|---|---|---|
| | | | h | % | | |
| Agte | Black bean, India | Not cooked | 24 | 31 | – | – |
| Agte | Black bean, India | Pressure cooked | 24 | 35 | – | – |
| Alonso | Kidney bean, Spain | Not cooked | 24 | 9 | 44 | 32 |
| Shimelis | Kidney bean, Ethiopia | Not cooked | 24 | 28–73 | 32–35 | – |
| Alonso | Kidney bean, Spain | Not cooked | 48 | 19 | 64 | 41 |
| Shimelis | Kidney bean, Ethiopia | Not cooked | 48 | 62–87 | 74–80 | – |
| Al-Numair | White bean, Sudan | Not cooked | 48 | 23–29 | – | 27–52 |

–, not reported
Soaking occurred as 1:3–1:5 seed:water ratio

## 4.8   Summary

Pulses provide many key minerals including iron, zinc and calcium which are particularly needed in LIC for adequate growth and development of children and adolescents, and women's health. However, bioavailability issues related to phytate and polyphenol (tannin) content of pulses may limit their usefulness as a mineral source unless appropriate processing of pulses is undertaken. These processes include soaking, germination, and fermentation. Determining whether processing has improved bioavailability may be done using in vivo or in vitro techniques, with many having limitations either in application to human nutrition or expense and logistics. Nevertheless with continued research including new ways of growing crops through biofortification, pulses will remain important contributors to mineral nutrition for many people globally.

## References

Ali M, Shuja MN, Zahoor M et al (2010) Phytic acid: how far have we come? Afr J Biotechnol 9:1551–1554

Bohn L, Meyer AS, Rasmussen SK (2008) Phytate: impact on environment and human nutrition. A challenge for molecular breeding. J Zhejiang Univ Sci B 9:165–191

Costa D, Almeida DA, Pissini SQ et al (2006) Chemical composition, dietary fibre and resistant starch contents of raw and cooked pea, common bean, chickpea and lentil legumes. Food Chem 94:327–330

Egli I, Davidsson L, Juillerat MA et al (2002) The influence of soaking and germination on the phytase activity and phytic acid content of grains and seeds potentially useful for complementary feeding. J Food Sci 67:3484–3488

Etcheverry P, Grusak MA, Fleige LE (2002) Application of in vitro bioaccessibility and bioavailability methods for calcium, carotenoids, folate, iron, magnesium, polyphenols, zinc, and vitamins B(6), B(12), D, and E. Front Physiol 3:317. https://doi.org/10.3389/fphys.2012.00317.

Fairweather-Tait S, Phillips I, Wortley G et al (2007) The use of solubility, dialyzability, and Caco-2 cell methods to predict iron bioavailability. Int J Vit Nutr Res 77:158–165

Fraga CG, Galleano M, Verstraeten SV et al (2010) Basic biochemical mechanisms behind the health benefits of polyphenols. Mol Asp Med 31:435–445

Fulgoni VL, Keast DR, Bailey RL et al (2011) Foods, fortificants, and supplements: where do Americans get their nutrients? J Nutr 141:1847–1854

García-Nebot MJ, Barberá R, Alegría A (2013) Iron and zinc bioavailability in Caco-2 cells: influence of caseinophosphopeptides. Food Chem 138:1298–1303

Gibson R (2011) Strategies for preventing multi-micronutrient deficiencies: a review of experiences with food-based approaches in developing countries, in combating micronutrient deficiencies. In: FAO and CABI, food-based approaches. p 7–27

Gibson R, Perlas L, Hotz C (2006) Improving the bioavailability of nutrients in plant foods at the household level. Proc Nutr Soc 65:160–168

Gibson RS, Bailey KB, Gibbs M et al (2010) A review of phytate, iron, zinc, and calcium concentrations in plant-based complementary foods used in low-income countries and implications for bioavailability. Food Nutr Bull 31(2 Suppl):S134–S146

Gibson RS, Raboy V, King JC (2018) Implications of phytate in plant-based foods for iron and zinc bioavailability, setting dietary requirements, and formulating programs and policies. Nutr Rev 76:793–804

Glahn R, Wortley GM, South PK et al (2002) Inhibition of iron uptake by phytic acid, tannic acid, and zncl2: studies using an in vitro digestion/Caco-2 cell model. J Agric Food Chem 50:390–395

Gupta R, Gangoliya S, Singh N (2015) Reduction of phytic acid and enhancement of bioavailable micronutrients in food grains. J Food Sci Technol 52:676–684

Haas JD, Luna SV, Lung'aho MG et al (2016) Consuming iron biofortified beans increases iron status in Rwandan women after 128 days in a randomized controlled feeding trial. J Nutr 146:1586–1592

Haileslassie H, Henry C, Tyler R (2016) Impact of household food processing strategies on antinutrient (phytate, tannin and polyphenol) contents of chickpeas (Cicerarietinum L.) and beans (*Phaseolus vulgaris* L.): a review. Int J Food Sci Technol 51:1947–1957

Henry C, Elabor- Idemudia P, Tsegaye G et al (2016) A gender framework for ensuring sensitivity to women's role in pulse production in southern Ethiopia. J Agric Sci 8:80–90

Hotz C (2005) Evidence for the usefulness of in vitro dialyzability, Caco-2 cell models, animal models, and algorithms to predict zinc bioavailability in humans. Int J Vit Nutr Res 75:423–435

Hotz C, Gibson R (2007) Traditional food processing and preparation practices to enhance the bioavailability of micronutrients in plant-based diets. J Nutr 137:1097–1100

Hurrell R (2002) Bioavailability – a time for reflection. Int J Vit Nutr Res 72:5–6

Hurrell R, Egli I (2010) Iron bioavailability and dietary reference values. Am J Clin Nutr 91:1461S–1467S

Kumar V, Sinha AK, Makkar HPS et al (2010) Dietary roles of phytate and phytase in human nutrition: a review. Food Chem 120:945–959

Lönnerdal B (2000) Dietary factors influencing zinc absorption. J Nutr 130:1378S–1383S

Lopez H, Leenhardt F, Coudray C et al (2002) Minerals and phytic acid interactions: is it real problem for human nutrition? Int J Food Sci Technol 37:727–739

Manach C, Scalbert A, Morand C et al (2004) Polyphenols: food sources and bioavailability. Am J Clin Nutr 79:727–747

Naczk M, Shahidi F (2004) Extraction and analysis of phenolics in food. J Chromatog A 1054:95–111

Nergiz C, Gökgöz E (2007) Effects of traditional cooking methods on some antinutrients and in vitro protein digestibility of dry bean varieties (*Phaseolus vulgaris* L.) grown in Turkey. Int J Food Sci Technol 42:868–873

Oatway L, Vasanthan T, Helm JH (2001) Phytic acid. Food Rev Int 17:419–431

Petry N, Egli I, Zeder C et al (2010) Polyphenols and phytic acid contribute to the low iron bioavailability from common beans in young women. J Nutr 140:1977–1982

Platel K, Srinivasan K (2016) Bioavailability of micronutrients from plant foods: an update. Crit Rev Food Sci Nutr 56:1608–1619

Pynaert I, Armah C, Fairweather-Tait S et al (2006) Iron solubility compared with in vitro digestion–Caco-2 cell culture method for the assessment of iron bioavailability in a processed and unprocessed complementary food for Tanzanian infants (6–12 months). Br J Nutr 95:721–726

Ray H, Bett K, Tar'an B et al (2014) Mineral micronutrient content of cultivars of field pea, chickpea, common bean, and lentil grown in Saskatchewan, Canada. Crop Sci 54:1698–1708

Ruel M, Alderman H (2013) Nutrition-sensitive interventions and programmes: how can they help to accelerate progress in improving maternal and child nutrition? Lancet 382:536–551

Sandberg A (2002) Bioavailability of minerals in legumes. Br J Nutr 88(S3):S281–S285

Siddiq M, Uebersax MA (2012) Dry beans and pulses production and consumption—an overview. In: Siddiq M, Uebersax MA (eds) Dry beans and pulses production, processing and nutrition. Blackwell Publishing Ltd, Oxford. https://doi.org/10.1002/9781118448298.ch1

Tako E, Vandenberg A, Thavarajah D et al (2011) Iron bioavailability in lentil based diets: studies in poultry and in vitro digestion/Caco-2 model. J Fed Am Soc Exp 25:607.8

Umeta M, West C, Fufa H (2005) Content of zinc, iron, calcium and their absorption inhibitors in foods commonly consumed in Ethiopia. J Food Comp Anal 18:803–817

Welch R, Graham R (2004) Breeding for micronutrients in staple food crops from a human nutrition perspective. J Exp Bot 55:353–364

Yun S, Habicht J, Miller DD et al (2004) An in vitro digestion/Caco-2 cell culture system accurately predicts the effects of ascorbic acid and polyphenolic compounds on iron bioavailability in humans. J Nutr 134:2717–2721

Zimmermann MB, Chaouki N, Hurrell RF (2005) Iron deficiency due to consumption of a habitual diet low in bioavailable iron: a longitudinal cohort study in Moroccan children. Am J Clin Nutr 81:115–121

# Chapter 5
# Pulses and Prevention and Management of Chronic Disease

Maryam Kazemi, Sam Buddemeyer, Claire Marie Fassett, Wendy M. Gans,
Kelly M. Johnston, Edda Lungu, Rachel L. Savelle, Pooja N. Tolani,
and Wendy J. Dahl

**Abstract** Pulses offer health benefits, and their favorable nutrient composition has the potential to improve diet quality. In developing countries, pulses improve nutrient intakes of populations at risk of consuming a diet of poor quality. In developed nations, pulses have been recommended as an integral component of a healthful dietary pattern. Epidemiological and interventional studies have provided insight into the benefits of pulse intake related to the prevention and management of chronic disease. This chapter discusses the evidence from human studies regarding the effects of pulse consumption on cardiovascular disease, hypertension, type 2 diabetes, and cancer risk. In addition, the novel application of a pulse-based diet in the management of polycystic ovary syndrome and the importance of pulses in maintaining the wellbeing of persons living with human immunodeficiency virus/acquired immune deficiency syndrome are highlighted. Emerging evidence related to pulse consumption, improved diet quality, and decreased burden of chronic disease support translational efforts to promote pulses as health-enhancing, sustainable food sources globally.

**Keywords** Pulses · Legumes · Cardiovascular disease · Diabetes · Polycystic ovarian syndrome · Cancer · HIV · Obesity · Satiety · Hypertension

M. Kazemi
Division of Nutritional Sciences, College of Human Ecology, Cornell University,
Ithaca, NY, USA
e-mail: mk2564@cornell.edu

S. Buddemeyer · C. M. Fassett · W. M. Gans · K. M. Johnston · E. Lungu · R. L. Savelle
P. N. Tolani · W. J. Dahl (✉)
Food Science and Human Nutrition Department, University of Florida, Gainesville, FL, USA
e-mail: seb132@ufl.edu; fassettc@ufl.edu; wgans5401@ufl.edu; kelmj@ufl.edu;
eddalungu@ufl.edu; rsavelle525@ufl.edu; pooja.tolani@ufl.edu; wdahl@ufl.edu

© Springer Nature Switzerland AG 2019
W. J. Dahl (ed.), *Health Benefits of Pulses*,
https://doi.org/10.1007/978-3-030-12763-3_5

## 5.1 Introduction

Pulses such as beans, peas, chickpeas, and lentils are inexpensive sources of protein and provide marginal nutrients critical to providing optimal nutrition to those experiencing food insecurity in developing countries. In developed countries, where protein intakes exceed requirements, pulses offer health benefits by decreasing the risk of chronic diseases, including obesity, and thus are recommended for inclusion in health-promoting dietary patterns (Health Canada 2007; Krebs-Smith et al. 2018; Panizza et al. 2018; Reedy et al. 2018).

A growing body of evidence supports the positive effects of pulses on diet quality (Mudryj et al. 2014). Pulses are the leading source of dry vegetable protein which contributes considerably to the essential amino acid requirements of the human diet (Iqbal et al. 2006; Mudryj et al. 2014). They contain approximately double the amount of protein found in whole-grain cereals such as wheat, and provide three times the protein content of rice. Pulses also are excellent sources of fiber, significant sources of vitamins and minerals, such as iron, zinc, folate, calcium, magnesium, and potassium, and are low in sodium.

Beyond their contribution to diet quality, pulse consumption may be associated with reduced risk of obesity (Papanikolaou and Fulgoni 2008), chronic diseases including cardiovascular disease (CVD) and type 2 diabetes (DM2) (Afshin et al. 2014; Zhu et al. 2015), and endocrine conditions such as polycystic ovarian syndrome (PCOS) (Kazemi et al. 2018). Accordingly, the favorable nutrient profile of pulse foods has led to investigations of their potential benefit in the prevention and management of chronic disease.

## 5.2 Weight Management

Obesity increases the risk of developing CVD, DM2, and some cancers (CDC 2017). Dietary and lifestyle modifications are well-established interventions for weight loss and are associated with reduced risk of chronic disease mortality (Ma et al. 2017). Healthy lifestyle behaviors, including health-promoting dietary patterns, are essential and integral strategies to achieve and sustain a healthy body weight. Observations from epidemiological studies suggest higher pulse consumption is associated with a lower risk of obesity. In a large global study of children, consumption of vegetables, nuts, and pulses was inversely associated with body mass index (BMI) (Wall et al. 2018). In adults, intake of plant proteins, including pulses and soy, were inversely associated with BMI and waist circumference (Lin et al. 2011). Data from the U.S. National Health and Nutrition Examination Survey (NHANES) shows that bean consumers have a lower body weight, smaller waist circumference, and a lower risk of obesity when compared to non-bean consumers (Papanikolaou and Fulgoni 2008).

Energy-restricted diets containing pulses have been shown to induce weight loss. A systematic review and meta-analysis of 21 trials including 940 overweight and obese, middle-aged adults concluded that pulse consumption may be effective in promoting weight loss (Kim et al. 2016). Participants who adhered to diets containing a median intake of approximately one serving (132 g/d) of pulses experienced a small, yet significant, weight reduction of 0.34 kg over a median study length of 6 weeks, when compared to subjects who consumed an isocaloric control diet. It has been proposed that a dietary pattern incorporating pulses may facilitate weight control through reduced absorption of macronutrients and increased satiety (Kim et al. 2016). The intervention trials discussed below support these hypotheses (McCrory et al. 2010; Mollard et al. 2012; Li et al. 2014).

## 5.2.1  Reduced Absorption of Energy from Macronutrients

Weight maintenance or weight loss associated with pulse consumption may be attributed to decreased digestion and absorption of macronutrients. Some of the starch in pulses is resistant starch (RS) (de Almeida Costa et al. 2006), and thus is not digested and absorbed in the small intestine. Pulse starch resistant to digestion is fermented in the colon which produces short chain fatty acids (SCFA). SCFA provide approximately 2 kcal/g of energy compared to the 4 kcal/g provided from digestible starch (Elia and Cummings 2007). However, it must be noted that RS content is dependent on cooking and processing. Thus, starch digestibility of processed pulses, including flours or canned foods, may be higher when compared to that of traditionally prepared pulse foods (Tovar et al. 1992). Intact cell walls with encapsulated starch recovered from small intestinal effluent (Noah et al. 1998) confirm that some of the starch in pulses is physically inaccessible to alpha-amylase. In addition to starch, some of the protein in pulses also may be resistant to digestion and would therefore provide less energy. The undigested or partially digested pulse protein also enters the colon, where it may be fermented by the gut microbiota (Yao et al. 2016).

## 5.2.2  Increased Satiety

The effect of pulse intake on satiety has been documented. A systematic review and meta-analysis including nine studies and 126 participants analyzed the effects of whole pulses on satiety and second meal food intake, defined as the food intake at a meal following the consumption of a test food or ingredient such as pulses. Incorporating 250–292 g of pulses into meals led to increased satiety compared to control diets (Li et al. 2014). Although pulses induced early satiation, they were not shown to decrease food intake at later meals. Likewise, McCrory et al. (2010)

concluded that the incorporation of dietary pulses into meals yielded higher satiety and decreased meal-time food intake.

A recent pilot study provided some insight into the mechanisms of satiety secondary to pulse consumption. The effect of naturally-occurring fiber in black beans was compared to those of added fiber, including cellulose and psyllium, and a no-fiber control meal on satiety in 12 individuals with metabolic syndrome (Reverri et al. 2017). After receiving isocaloric meals, subjects who consumed whole black beans had a higher postprandial cholecystokinin and peptide YY, and lower insulin concentrations, when compared to their counterparts who consumed added fiber or no fiber. The observations support the benefits of whole bean intake on appetite-regulating hormonal responses in individuals with metabolic syndrome.

Pulses may induce satiety via their favorable macronutrient profile. Pulses are high in protein and fiber, and contain complex carbohydrates that are slowly digested (McCrory et al. 2010). High fiber foods are thought to increase satiety, in part due to an increased chewing time, stimulating early satiety signals (Howarth et al. 2001). Further, pulses contain soluble fiber that may contribute to luminal viscosity leading to a reduced rate of gastric emptying and less physical contact of nutrients with intestinal villi, thereby decreasing the rate of food absorption through the digestive system (Howarth et al. 2001). In addition, increased satiety secondary to pulse consumption has been attributed to their high protein content through established mechanisms (Lejeune et al. 2006). Together, the satiating effects of pulses appear to be multifactorial and related to their slow digestibility and favorable nutritional composition, including protein, starch, and fiber.

## 5.3   Cancer

The Second World Cancer Research Fund/American Institute for Cancer Research Expert Report recommends the consumption of "relatively unprocessed cereals (grains) and/or pulses, and other foods that are natural sources of dietary fiber, to contribute to a population average daily consumption of 25 g of non-starch polysaccharides" (Wiseman 2008). The inclusion of mostly plant-based foods, including pulses, while limiting meat, especially processed meat, in the diet is recommended (WCRF n.d.).

Previous studies support the association between higher intakes of pulses and a decreased risk of colorectal cancer (Zhu et al. 2015; Wang et al. 2013). Prospective studies have shown an inverse association between pulse intake and the risk of prostate cancer (Diallo et al. 2016). Cohort studies have also demonstrated a dose-response reduction in the risk of prostate cancer with an increment in pulse intake (Li and Mao 2017). The consumption of beans has been associated with a lower risk of breast cancer in women (Velie et al. 2005). The 'Four Corner Breast Cancer Study' found that the incidence of breast cancer among ethnic groups that consumed high amounts of pulses was lower compared to their counterparts who consumed low amounts (Murtaugh et al. 2008).

Pulses contain a variety of constituents which may help to reduce cancer risk if consumed in sufficient quantities (Mathers 2002). Resistant starch, non-starch polysaccharides, oligosaccharides, folate, selenium, zinc, and bioactive macroconstituents such as protease inhibitors, phytosterols, lectins, phytochemicals, saponins, tannins, and phytates are purported to have anti-carcinogenic effects. The anticarcinogenic effects of pulses have been attributed to mechanisms associated with digestion, fermentation by gut microbiota, repair of DNA damage, and apoptosis of damaged cells (Mathers 2002). Of note, the nutritive components may have a beneficial effect only in the event of deficiency.

Collectively, the current evidence suggests a higher intake of pulses is associated with reduced risk of various cancers. Further high-quality research is required to evaluate the potential benefits of pulse consumption on the prevention and prognosis of cancer.

## 5.4 Cardiovascular Disease

Cardiovascular disease is a leading cause of death worldwide and is associated with risk factors such as diabetes, dyslipidemia, obesity, aging, and hypertension (HTN) (USDHHS 2017). Prospective and retrospective studies have shown negative associations between pulse intake and the risk of CVD (Afshin et al. 2014). Recent data from the Prospective Urban Rural Epidemiology (PURE) found legume (including pulse) consumption to be inversely associated with "cardiovascular disease, myocardial infarction, cardiovascular mortality, non-cardiovascular mortality, and total mortality" (Miller et al. 2017).

Interventions for the prevention of CVD typically focus on modifiable risk factors. Some of these factors, specifically body weight, HTN, hyperlipidemia, and hyperglycemia, can be modified through dietary interventions. Evidence suggests that increased consumption of pulses can improve these modifiable risk factors and may reduce the risk for CVD. Dietary pulses fit well into health-promoting dietary patterns, such as the Mediterranean and Dietary Approach to Stop Hypertension (DASH) and contribute plant protein, fiber, and potassium – properties that yield a potential cardiovascular protective effect by lowering cholesterol and regulating blood pressure.

### 5.4.1 Serum Cholesterol

A meta-analysis examining 11 clinical trials with 187 participants consuming an average of 110 g of pulses (dry beans) reported reduction of total serum cholesterol reduction by 7%, low-density lipoprotein cholesterol (LDL-C) by 6%, and serum triacylglycerols by 17%, while maintaining high-density lipoprotein cholesterol (HDL-C) levels (Anderson and Major 2002). A more recent meta-analysis of ten randomized controlled trials (RCTs) of at least 3 weeks in length compared non-soy legume diets (mixed legumes, whole chickpeas, beans, and peas) to similar total energy and macronutrient controls (Bazzano et al. 2011). A total of 268 participants with high, borderline high, and normal cholesterol levels were represented, and blood lipid changes were measured during the intervention and control (substituted with a wheat-based or canned vegetable) periods. Total cholesterol and LDL-C were significantly lower with the intervention, while the decrease seen in triglyceride level was non-significant. A meta-analysis of 26 RCTs analyzed 1037 participants (Ha et al. 2014). Eight trials selected patients with hyperlipidemia, three included patients with normal lipid profiles, and the remaining 15 trials included both normal- and hyperlipidemia. The authors concluded that a median intake of 130 g/d of dietary pulses (beans, peas, chickpeas, lentils, and mixed, in flour or whole format) lowered LDL-C significantly when compared with the isocaloric control. Mean improvements in non-HDL cholesterol also favored the increase in dietary pulse intake. An intervention trial found that pulses used in combination with whole grains provide potential to improve cardiovascular-associated risk biomarkers in healthy women (Tovar et al. 2014). A combination of beans and whole barley significantly decreased total cholesterol and LDL-C, and reduced apolipoprotein B (apoB), blood pressure, and cardiovascular disease risk in these women. The positive effects of pulse consumption on total cholesterol and LDL-C were further supported by a 2-month, pulse-based diet trial (i.e., two servings per day of pulses, or 150 g/d dry weight) which reduced total cholesterol and LDL-C-cholesterol by 8%, and improved body composition (i.e., reduced body fat %) in men and women over 50 years of age, an age-group with an increased risk of CVD (Abeysekara et al. 2012).

Cardiovascular risk reduction through modulating lipid profile, inflammation, and oxidative activities through various compounds present in pulses such as fiber, monounsaturated fatty acids and polyunsaturated fatty acids, phenols, vitamin E, carotenoids, and phospholipids, have been delineated through epidemiological studies and clinical trials (Souza et al. 2015). The cholesterol lowering effects of pulses have been attributed to their insoluble fiber content, which binds bile acids or cholesterol during the intraluminal formation of micelles, thereby reducing the cholesterol content of liver cells, up-regulating the LDL-C receptors, and increasing the clearance of LDL-C (Brown et al. 1999). However, increased bile acid excretion may not be sufficient to account for the observed cholesterol reduction (Pilch 1987). Fermentation of dietary fiber in the colon leads to the exogenous synthesis of SCFA (e.g. acetate, butyrate, propionate) (Koh et al. 2016) which provide a minor amount of energy but are essential signalling molecules involved in improving lipid metabolism (Koh et al. 2016). The microbial conversion of dietary fiber into functionally relevant metabolites has been proposed to improve host gut microbiota composition and protection from metabolic disease, through improved immunity, decreased hepatic synthesis of cholesterol and glucose (Kishimoto et al. 1995; van Bennekum et al. 2005; Chibbar et al. 2010) and increased insulin sensitivity (Schneeman 1987; Koh et al. 2016).

## 5.4.2 Hypertension

Hypertension is another modifiable risk factor and therapeutic target in the prevention of CVD. In addition to improving blood lipid concentrations, pulses have been shown to improve blood pressure. Jayalath et al. (2014) performed a meta-analysis on eight isocaloric trials including 554 participants, and showed pulse consumption (~162 g/d) over 10 weeks reduced mean arterial blood pressure by −0.75 mmHg in middle-aged subjects with or without HTN. The authors reported that when pulses were exchanged isocalorically for other foods, both systolic blood pressure and mean arterial blood pressure were lowered significantly.

Pulses may confer blood pressure-lowering effects by increasing dietary intakes of dietary fiber, plant protein, potassium, and magnesium, as well as decreasing sodium intake through established mechanisms (Jee et al. 2002; Altorf-van der Kuil et al. 2010; Aburto et al. 2013; Tielemans et al. 2013; Mudryj et al. 2014).

## 5.5 Diabetes

A systematic review and meta-analysis of cohort studies assessing legume intake (including pulses) and risk of DM2 was not conclusive (Afshin et al. 2014). The report describes two cohort studies. One followed 64,191 middle-aged Chinese women without a history of DM2, cancer, or CVD for an average of 4.6 years (Villegas et al. 2008). The study analyzed bean, lentil, peanut, pea, and soybean intake. Beans, lentils, and peas were grouped as "other legumes" and were analyzed separately. Average consumption of "other legumes" was 15.5 g per day. The multivariate-adjusted relative risk of DM2 incidence was inversely associated with "other legume" intake by quintile. The lowest and highest "other legume" intake quintiles were 5.6 g/day (relative risk (RR): 1.00) and 37.1 g/day (RR: 0.76; 95% CI: 0.64–0.90), respectively. The authors concluded that consumption of "other legumes" was significantly associated with a decreased risk of DM2 when comparing the upper quintile to the lower quintile. The second cohort study examined the link between grains, vegetables, fruits, and legumes and the incidence of DM2 in 35,988 women in Iowa (Meyer et al. 2000). After the 6-year follow up, the study concluded that neither the overall intake of, nor the fiber derived from legumes was related to DM2 risk. Total intake of mature beans ranged from <1.5 servings/week to >4.5 servings/week (1 serving = 100 g). The intake of fiber from legumes in the study was very low, ranging from <0.31 g/day in the lowest intake quartile to >1.21 g/day in the highest quartile. The authors concluded that the intake might have been too small to show an effect on DM2 risk. When the two cohort studies were pooled in the meta-analysis, legume consumption was not significantly associated with the incidence of DM2. The analysis did not differentiate between all legumes and pulses separately. There are obvious limitations to the studies in that both included women only and both utilized food frequency questionnaires that rely on the accuracy of self-reporting. Using the Grading of Recommendations, Assessment, Development, and Evaluation tool to evaluate the strength of the evidence, Viguiliouk et al. (2017) rated the evidence for the relationship between legume intake and risk of DM2 as low. While adherence to a priori dietary patterns that are rich in pulses, such as the Mediterranean and DASH dietary patterns, have been associated with a decreased risk of DM2 (Salas-Salvado et al. 2014), it is not possible to discern causality from the associations or the specific role of pulses. The link between pulse consumption and the risk of DM2 remains to be confirmed through prospective research.

### 5.5.1 Glycemic Response

Due to the well-established link between chronically elevated glucose levels and organ and nerve damage, as well as an increased risk for CVD, achieving glycemic control is one of the primary goals in the medical management of persons with diabetes (Cheng 2013). A review of the studies above examining the effects of pulse consumption on health outcomes related to the management of diabetes, shows strong evidence for their role in reducing blood lipids (Ha et al. 2014) and regulating body weight (Kim et al. 2016). Pulse consumption also may be beneficial on markers of glycemic control, including postprandial glucose levels, insulin responses, and hemoglobin A1c (HbA1c) (Sievenpiper et al. 2009).

Pulses contain a mixture of dietary fibers (Tosh and Yada 2010) which contribute to gastrointestinal luminal viscosity, fecal bulking, and fermentability. Glucose-lowering effects have been attributed to viscous, soluble fibers, but there also is evidence for the effectiveness of resistant starch in lowering postprandial glucose. Viscous, soluble fiber may act to improve glucose control by delaying gastric emptying and delaying, or possibly decreasing, the absorption of glucose (Viguiliouk et al. 2017). Both acute and long-term studies have shown reduced postprandial glucose and insulin response following dietary intake of pulses (Jenkins et al. 2012). It is suggested that this occurs because they slow absorption in the small intestine, in turn lowering the overall glycemic index (GI) of the meal (Nestel et al. 2004; Torsdottir et al. 1989; Mollard et al. 2012). Similarly, studies using RS were found to significantly lower postprandial glucose levels and increase insulin sensitivity (Fuentes-Zaragoza et al. 2010; Kwak et al. 2012; Jenkins et al. 2002). This suggests that the effect is enhanced when RS is combined with soluble fiber, lending evidence to a synergistic effect that supports the consumption of whole foods with a mix of fiber types over supplementation with isolated fiber sources (Behall et al. 2006).

A meta-analysis of randomized controlled trials found that low-GI diets reduced HbA1c by 0.43% points more than did their high-GI counterparts (Brand-Miller et al. 2003) and that higher fiber diets play a role in lowering postprandial blood glucose and insulin levels (Fuller et al. 2016). When examining the postprandial effects of pulse foods compared to controls (e.g. rice, grains, glucose, isolated fibers, and potatoes), the majority of studies found significant reductions in postprandial glucose relative to controls (Jenkins et al. 2012; Shams et al. 2010). Meta-analyses of randomized controlled trials have determined that pulses lower insulin and fasting blood glucose levels as well as HbA1c (Sievenpiper et al. 2009). The meta-analyses included trial interventions of pulses alone, pulses as part of a low-GI diet, and pulses as part of a high fiber diet. Beneficial reductions were seen across all three categories of interventions, but effects were most pronounced when pulses were coupled with low-GI and high fiber diets. The U.S. Food and Drug Administration requires a clinically meaningful threshold of a reduction of $\geq 0.3\%$ in HbA1c for a new diabetic drug to be approved (USFDA 2008). When the standardized mean difference was used to calculate the average absolute reduction in HbA1c for pulses included as part of a low-GI diet, the absolute reduction was 0.5%, indicating that an overall low-GI diet supplemented with dietary pulses can exceed the effects of some diabetic drugs with regard to improvements in HbA1c.

DM2 is commonly accompanied by the co-morbidities of dyslipidemia and obesity, both of which are known to increase the risk for CVD. Multiple meta-analyses have shown improvements in blood lipid levels with the incorporation of pulses in the diet and support their use in the management of hyperlipidemia in individuals with DM2 (Anderson and Major 2002; Bazzano et al. 2011; Ha et al. 2014). Pulse consumption also has been shown to regulate body weight and reduce obesity risk through improved satiety and subsequent reduction in food intake (Jenkins et al. 2012; Kim et al. 2016). Long-term consumption of pulses has been shown to modulate glucose and insulin responses of patients with DM2, and improve weight control by reducing appetite and energy intake (McCrory et al. 2010). However, the isolated effect of pulses on glycemic response in DM2 is less clear. Many trials have classified pulses as a whole grain, thus interpretation of the isolated positive effects of pulses is difficult to ascertain (Jacobs et al. 1998; Jang et al. 2001). Further, the reported low intake and duration of pulse consumption were likely too small to claim that pulse consumption reflected a genuine effect on DM2 control. Nevertheless, "there is strong evidence to suggest eating a variety of whole grains and legumes is beneficial in the treatment and management of diabetes" (Venn and Mann 2004). Theoretically, some unprocessed whole grains share the nutritional profile of pulses including a high fiber content and lower GI. However, it is important to investigate the isolated effects of pulses on DM2 management. Collectively, the available evidence provides support for the beneficial role of pulses in the management of diabetes and prevention and management of its comorbidities. However, additional research is required to conclude the optimal type and dose of pulses that would improve DM2 outcomes.

## 5.6 Polycystic Ovary Syndrome

Polycystic ovary syndrome (PCOS) is a common endocrine and metabolic disorder and the leading cause of anovulatory infertility among reproductive-age women worldwide, with a prevalence of up to 18% (Carmina and Lobo 1999; March et al. 2010). In addition to infertility, PCOS is associated with profound metabolic abnormalities which contribute to increased rates of long-term morbidity, including DM2 and CVD (Carmina and Lobo 1999; Diamanti-Kandarakis and Dunaif 2012; Wild et al. 2010). Women with PCOS exhibit insulin resistance and hyperinsulinemia, with associated metabolic aberrations including dysglycemia, dyslipidemia, HTN, and abdominal adiposity (Diamanti-Kandarakis and Dunaif 2012; Teede et al. 2018).

Lifestyle modifications comprised of dietary, exercise, and behavioral therapies have been recommended as first-line approaches in the management of PCOS (Azziz et al. 2006; Moran et al. 2011; Teede et al. 2011). However, according to the recent international guidelines for the assessment and management of PCOS, there is limited evidence regarding a specific dietary composition which is better than others for improving PCOS health outcomes (Teede et al. 2018). Controversy surrounds the optimal diet composition to mediate favorable health benefits for women with PCOS. Previous RCTs focused exhaustively on the benefits of weight loss for improving PCOS health outcomes in obese or overweight women (Becker et al. 2015; Mehrabani et al. 2012; Stamets et al. 2004; Thomson et al. 2008) through rapid, short-term energy restriction per se, which is less attainable and sustainable. There is a lack of evidence on favorable dietary compositions, independent of energy restriction, to mediate advantageous health benefits in women with PCOS.

Pulses have received insufficient attention in the context of PCOS research. In North America, pulse consumption is low and neglected despite its health benefits (DHHS and USDA n.d.; USDA 2016). Previous work has provided some insights into the long-term benefits of pulse consumption on various health outcomes in non-PCOS populations which share metabolic abnormalities with women with PCOS (Abeysekara et al. 2012; Ha et al. 2014; McCrory et al. 2010; Mudryj et al. 2014). Long-term pulse consumption has been associated with positive cardiometabolic effects such as lowering postprandial blood glucose and insulin concentrations, and decreasing hypercholesterolemia, blood pressure, and obesity (Abeysekara et al. 2012; Ha et al. 2014; McCrory et al. 2010; Sievenpiper et al. 2009). Due to the overlapping pathophysiological underpinnings between PCOS and DM2, it is plausible that adherence to a pulse-rich diet alleviates systemic insulin resistance and cardiometabolic risk factors, and subsequently polycystic ovarian morphology and ovulation dysfunction in women with PCOS. Further, many women with PCOS are overweight and obese (Apridonidze et al. 2005; Gambineri et al. 2002; Glueck et al. 2003, 2009; Wright et al. 2004; Yildiz et al. 2008). Women with PCOS have difficulties with weight loss, in part due to abnormal insulin and glucose homeostasis (Motta 2012; Lim et al. 2007, 2013).

Pulses can mediate satiety and weight management due to their high fiber content, moderate energy density, and complex and slowly digestible carbohydrate composition (Li et al. 2014; Marinangeli and Jones 2012; McCrory et al. 2010; Mollard et al. 2012). However, few RCTs have examined the effects of pulse consumption on the health outcomes in women with PCOS. In a multi-dimensional RCT without a prescribed energy-restricted protocol (Kazemi et al. 2018), the benefits of a pulse-based, low-GI diet, which included split-peas, lentils, beans, and chickpeas, over the National Cholesterol Education Program Adult Treatment Panel

III Therapeutic Lifestyle Changes (TLC) diet (NCEP 2002) on the cardiometabolic health of women with PCOS were demonstrated. Participating women received education and health counseling about PCOS and the benefits of lifestyle modification, and were encouraged to exercise as a standard of care. Specifically, a pulse-based diet was more effective for improving insulin sensitivity, dyslipidemia, and diastolic blood pressure when compared to the TLC diet. The improved lipid profiles were noteworthy, as the control TLC diet is recommended to elicit hypocholesterolemic effects in people at risk for CVD and DM2 (NCEP 2002). By extrapolation, a risk reduction of 8–12% for future major cardiovascular events following the consumption of a pulse-based diet compared to the TLC diet was estimated (CTT et al. 2012; Manson et al. 1992). It has been postulated that the hypocholesterolemic effects of the pulse-based diet stem primarily from its high fiber content, followed by decreased intakes of dietary cholesterol and *trans* fats, higher consumption of low-GI foods and a subsequent increase in insulin sensitivity, and higher intakes of protective nutrients such as minerals, folate, and antioxidant compounds such as tannins, flavonoids, polyphenols, phytates, lectins, and saponins (Anderson and Major 2002; Brown et al. 1999; Ludwig 2002; Mudryj et al. 2014). The observed decrease in insulin resistance in women with PCOS in the pulse-based diet group may be due to slower digestibility and modified glycemic response secondary to pulse consumption (Mudryj et al. 2014; Sievenpiper et al. 2009). However, the direct effect of pulses on glucoregulation, recommended dosage of pulses, and optimal duration of pulse consumption needed to prevent insulin resistance, impaired glucose tolerance, and DM2 is less clear and warrant further investigation.

Emerging evidence supports a novel view concerning the positive effects of pulse consumption on PCOS cardiometabolic health. High-quality, longitudinal RCTs are needed to elucidate the effects of pulse consumption on CVD risk, weight management, and reproductive health outcomes in women with PCOS across a range of body mass index, age, and PCOS phenotypes. Attempts should be made to educate women with PCOS about the health benefits of pulse consumption and to help them understand how to incorporate pulses in their diet. There is likely to be greater long-term adherence to consumption of pulses and a higher probability for long-term health improvements when women are educated on incorporating low-GI, nutrient-rich pulses into their everyday diet in ways suited to their palate.

## 5.7  Human Immunodeficiency Virus/Acquired Immunodeficiency Syndrome

Human immunodeficiency virus (HIV) and acquired immunodeficiency syndrome (AIDS) are prevalent in many developing countries and associated with poor nutritional status. Compromised nutritional status secondary to HIV/AIDS-related complications can further exacerbate the progression of the disease and increased mortality rates, despite antiretroviral treatment (Aberman et al. 2014). In HIV/AIDS affected households in some African countries, dietary diversity poses a great challenge due to the dependency on starchy foods (Bukusuba et al. 2010; Ezechi et al. 2016) with little animal-sourced foods. Incorporating pulse foods can diversify diets and improve protein intake, thereby improving the nutritional status of individuals living with HIV/AIDS. Their nutritional benefits and low cost make pulses an important contributor to minimizing or eliminating hunger and poor health due to HIV/AIDS (Odendo et al. 2011). Pulses can be incorporated as ingredients in other foods to make them more nutrient dense and potentially decreasing the progression rate of HIV to AIDS. Pulse foods were generally acceptable to Kenyan HIV-positive women and can be used to improve the nutritional intakes of persons living with HIV (Hong et al. 2013). A study in Tanzanian HIV-infected children who were fed bean-fortified products reported improved mid-upper-arm circumference, and their fat stores and blood hemoglobin levels also improved compared to children who consumed cereal products alone (Nnyepi et al. 2015). Many persons living with HIV/AIDS in developed countries are at risk for food insecurity, undernutrition, chronic low-grade inflammation, and associated cardiometabolic chronic disease risk (Willig et al. 2018). Pulses can serve as healthy and affordable foods with potential to improve diet quality and food security in underprivileged, HIV/AIDS-infected populations worldwide.

## 5.8 Summary

Consumption of pulses can improve overall diet quality and reduce the risk of several chronic diseases. Emerging research evidence supports the position that pulses have positive health benefits on the prevention and management of cardiometabolic disease and obesity across age, ethnic, BMI, and sex groups. Recent observations provide new insights into the benefits of pulse consumption on health outcomes in under-studies populations with compromised endocrine and immunodeficient conditions including PCOS and HIV/AIDS. The mechanisms through which pulse consumption can improve host gut microbiota composition, immunity, metabolic profile, and inflammatory response is yet to be explored. Further high-quality longitudinal studies are required to address the barriers toward pulse consumption. Pulse producers need to invest in research to examine opportunities to increase pulse consumption, including the adaptation of pulses into daily eating patterns in North America and promoting the nutritional benefits of pulses. Globally, increased awareness of the nutritional benefits of pulses, as part of sustainable food production is warranted to improve diet quality, promote health, and decrease food insecurity and hunger.

# References

Aberman NL, Rawat R, Drimie S et al (2014) Food security and nutrition interventions in response to the AIDS epidemic: assessing global action and evidence. AIDS Behav 18(Suppl 5): S554–S565

Abeysekara S, Chilibeck PD, Vatanparast H et al (2012) A pulse-based diet is effective for reducing total and LDL-cholesterol in older adults. Br J Nutr 108(Suppl S1):S103–S110

Aburto NJ, Hanson S, Gutierrez H et al (2013) Effect of increased potassium intake on cardiovascular risk factors and disease: systematic review and meta-analyses. BMJ 346:f1378

Afshin A, Micha R, Khatibzadeh S et al (2014) Consumption of nuts and legumes and risk of incident ischemic heart disease, stroke, and diabetes: a systematic review and meta-analysis. Am J Clin Nutr 100:278–288

de Almeida Costa GE, da Silva Q-MK, Pissini Machado Reis SM et al (2006) Chemical composition, dietary fibre and resistant starch contents of raw and cooked pea, common bean, chickpea and lentil legumes. Food Chem 94:327–330

Altorf-van der Kuil W, Engberink MF, Brink EJ et al (2010) Dietary protein and blood pressure: a systematic review. PLoS One 5:e12102

Anderson JW, Major AW (2002) Pulses and lipaemia, short- and long-term effect: potential in the prevention of cardiovascular disease. Br J Nutr 88(Suppl 3):S263–S271

Apridonidze T, Essah PA, Luorno MJ et al (2005) Prevalence and characteristics of the metabolic syndrome in women with polycystic ovary syndrome. J Clin Endocrinol Metab 90:1929–1935

Azziz R, Carmina E, Dewailly D et al (2006) Positions statement: criteria for defining polycystic ovary syndrome as a predominantly hyperandrogenic syndrome: an androgen excess society guideline. J Clin Endocrinol Metab 91:4237–4245

Bazzano LA, Thompson AM, Tees MT et al (2011) Non-soy legume consumption lowers cholesterol levels: a meta-analysis of randomized controlled trials. Nutr Metab Cardiovasc Dis 21:94–103

Becker GF, Passos EP, Moulin CC (2015) Short-term effects of a hypocaloric diet with low glycemic index and low glycemic load on body adiposity, metabolic variables, ghrelin, leptin, and pregnancy rate in overweight and obese infertile women: a randomized controlled trial. Am J Clin Nutr 102:1365–1372

Behall KM, Scholfield DJ, Hallfrisch JG et al (2006) Consumption of both resistant starch and beta-glucan improves postprandial plasma glucose and insulin in women. Diabetes Care 29:976–981

van Bennekum AM, Nguyen DV, Schulthess G et al (2005) Mechanisms of cholesterol-lowering effects of dietary insoluble fibres: relationships with intestinal and hepatic cholesterol parameters. Br J Nutr 94:331–337

Brand-Miller J, Hayne S, Petocz P et al (2003) Low-glycemic index diets in the management of diabetes: a meta-analysis of randomized controlled trials. Diabetes Care 26:2261–2267

Brown L, Rosner B, Willett WW et al (1999) Cholesterol-lowering effects of dietary fiber: a meta-analysis. Am J Clin Nutr 69:30–42

Bukusuba J, Kikafunda JK, Whitehead RG (2010) Nutritional knowledge, attitudes, and practices of women living with HIV in eastern Uganda. J Health Popul Nutr 28:182

Carmina E, Lobo RA (1999) Polycystic ovary syndrome (PCOS): arguably the most common endocrinopathy is associated with significant morbidity in women. J Clin Endocrinol Metab 84:1897–1899

Center for Disease Control (CDC) (2017) Overweight and Obesity. https://www.cdc.gov/obesity/adult/causes.html. Accessed 2 Dec 2018

Cheng AY (2013) Canadian Diabetes Association 2013 clinical practice guidelines for the prevention and management of diabetes in Canada. Introduction Can J Diabetes 37(Suppl 1):S1–S3

Chibbar RN, Ambigaipalan P, Hoover R (2010) Review: molecular diversity in pulse seed starch and complex carbohydrates and its role in human nutrition and health. Cereal Chem 87:342–352

Cholesterol Treatment Trialists' (CTT) Collaborators, Mihaylova B, Emberson J et al (2012) The effects of lowering LDL cholesterol with statin therapy in people at low risk of vascular disease: meta-analysis of individual data from 27 randomised trials. Lancet 380(9841):581–590

Diallo A, Deschasaux M, Galan P et al (2016) Associations between fruit, vegetable and legume intakes and prostate cancer risk: results from the prospective supplementation en Vitamines et Mineraux Antioxydants (SU.VI.MAX) cohort. Br J Nutr 115:1579–1585

Diamanti-Kandarakis E, Dunaif A (2012) Insulin resistance and the polycystic ovary syndrome revisited: an update on mechanisms and implications. Endocr Rev 33:981–1030

Elia M, Cummings JH (2007) Physiological aspects of energy metabolism and gastrointestinal effects of carbohydrates. Eur J Clin Nutr 61(Suppl 1):S40–S74

Ezechi L, Brai B, Osifeso G et al (2016) Nutritional knowledge, attitude and practices of women living with HIV/AIDS in Lagos Southwest, Nigeria. Mal J Nutr 22:1–15

Fuentes-Zaragoza E, Riquelme-Navarrete M, Sánchez-Zapata E et al (2010) Resistant starch as functional ingredient: a review. Food Res Int 43:931–942

Fuller S, Beck E, Salman H et al (2016) New horizons for the study of dietary fiber and health: a review. Plant Foods Hum Nutr 71:1–12

Gambineri A, Pelusi C, Vicennati V et al (2002) Obesity and the polycystic ovary syndrome. Int J Obes Relat Metab Disord 26:883–897

Glueck CJ, Papanna R, Wang P et al (2003) Incidence and treatment of metabolic syndrome in newly referred women with confirmed polycystic ovarian syndrome. Metabolism 52:908–915

Glueck CJ, Morrison JA, Goldenberg N et al (2009) Coronary heart disease risk factors in adult premenopausal white women with polycystic ovary syndrome compared with a healthy female population. Metabolism 58:714–721

Ha V, Sievenpiper JL, de Souza RJ et al (2014) Effect of dietary pulse intake on established therapeutic lipid targets for cardiovascular risk reduction: a systematic review and meta-analysis of randomized controlled trials. CMAJ 186:E252–E262

Health Canada (2007) Eating well with Canada's food guide. http://www.hc-sc.gc.ca/fn-an/alt_formats/hpfb-dgpsa/pdf/food-guide-aliment/print_eatwell_bienmang-eng.pdf. Accessed 13 Dec 2018

Hong SY, Hendricks KM, Wanke C et al (2013) Development of a nutrient-dense food supplement for HIV-infected women in rural Kenya using qualitative and quantitative research methods. Public Health Nutr 16:721–729

Howarth NC, Saltzman E, Roberts SB (2001) Dietary fiber and weight regulation. Nutr Rev 59:129–139

Iqbal A, Khalil IA, Ateeq N et al (2006) Nutritional quality of important food legumes. Food Chem 97:331–335

Jacobs D, Meyer KA, Kushi LH et al (1998) Whole-grain intake may reduce the risk of ischemic heart disease death in postmenopausal women: the Iowa Women's Health Study. Am J Clin Nutr 68:248–257

Jang Y, Lee JH, Kim OY et al (2001) Consumption of whole grain and legume powder reduces insulin demand, lipid peroxidation, and plasma homocysteine concentrations in patients with coronary artery disease randomized controlled clinical trial. Arterioscler Thromb Vasc Biol 21:2065–2071

Jayalath VH, de Souza RJ, Sievenpiper JL et al (2014) Effect of dietary pulses on blood pressure: a systematic review and meta-analysis of controlled feeding trials. Am J Hypertens 27:56–64

Jee SH, Miller ER, Guallar E et al (2002) The effect of magnesium supplementation on blood pressure: a meta-analysis of randomized clinical trials. Am J Hypertens 15:691–696

Jenkins DJ, Kendall CW, Augustin LS et al (2002) High-complex carbohydrate or lente carbohydrate foods? Am J Med 113(Suppl 9B):30s–37s

Jenkins DJ, Kendall CW, Augustin LS et al (2012) Effect of legumes as part of a low glycemic index diet on glycemic control and cardiovascular risk factors in type 2 diabetes mellitus: a randomized controlled trial. Arch Intern Med 172:1653–1660

Kazemi M, McBreairty LE, Chizen DR et al (2018) A comparison of a pulse-based diet and the therapeutic lifestyle changes diet in combination with exercise and health counselling on the cardio-metabolic risk profile in women with polycystic ovary syndrome: a randomized controlled trial. Nutrients 10:1387

Kim SJ, de Souza RJ, Choo VL et al (2016) Effects of dietary pulse consumption on body weight: a systematic review and meta-analysis of randomized controlled trials. Am J Clin Nutr 103:1213–1223

Kishimoto Y, Wakabayashi S, Takeda H (1995) Hypocholesterolemic effect of dietary fiber: relation to intestinal fermentation and bile acid excretion. J Nutr Sci Vitaminol 41:151–161

Koh A, De Vadder F, Kovatcheva-Datchary P et al (2016) From dietary fiber to host physiology: short-chain fatty acids as key bacterial metabolites. Cell 165:1332–1345

Krebs-Smith SM, Pannucci TE, Subar AF et al (2018) Update of the healthy eating index: HEI-2015. J Acad Nutr Diet 118:1591–1602

Kwak JH, Paik JK, Kim HI et al (2012) Dietary treatment with rice containing resistant starch improves markers of endothelial function with reduction of postprandial blood glucose and oxidative stress in patients with prediabetes or newly diagnosed type 2 diabetes. Atherosclerosis 224:457–464

Lejeune MP, Westerterp KR, Adam TC et al (2006) Ghrelin and glucagon-like peptide 1 concentrations, 24-h satiety, and energy and substrate metabolism during a high-protein diet and measured in a respiration chamber. Am J Clin Nutr 83:89–94

Li J, Mao QQ (2017) Legume intake and risk of prostate cancer: a meta-analysis of prospective cohort studies. Oncotarget 8:44776–44784

Li SS, Kendall CW, de Souza RJ et al (2014) Dietary pulses, satiety and food intake: a systematic review and meta-analysis of acute feeding trials. Obesity (Silver Spring) 22:1773–1780

Lim SS, Clifton PM, Noakes M et al (2007) Obesity management in women with polycystic ovary syndrome. Women Health (London, England) 3:73–86

Lim S, Norman R, Davies M et al (2013) The effect of obesity on polycystic ovary syndrome: a systematic review and meta-analysis. Obes Rev 14:95–109

Lin Y, Bolca S, Vandevijvere S et al (2011) Plant and animal protein intake and its association with overweight and obesity among the Belgian population. Br J Nutr 105:1106–1116

Ludwig DS (2002) The glycemic index: physiological mechanisms relating to obesity, diabetes, and cardiovascular disease. JAMA 287:2414–2423

Ma C, Avenell A, Bolland M et al (2017) Effects of weight loss interventions for adults who are obese on mortality, cardiovascular disease, and cancer: systematic review and meta-analysis. BMJ 359:j4849

Manson JE, Tosteson H, Ridker PM et al (1992) The primary prevention of myocardial infarction. New Eng J Med 326:1406–1416

March WA, Moore VM, Willson KJ et al (2010) The prevalence of polycystic ovary syndrome in a community sample assessed under contrasting diagnostic criteria. Hum Reprod 25:544–551

Marinangeli CPF, Jones PJH (2012) Pulse grain consumption and obesity: effects on energy expenditure, substrate oxidation, body composition, fat deposition and satiety. Br J Nutr 108:S46–S51

Mathers JC (2002) Pulses and carcinogenesis: potential for the prevention of colon, breast and other cancers. Br J Nutr 88(Suppl 3):273–279

McCrory MA, Hamaker BR, Lovejoy JC et al (2010) Pulse consumption, satiety, and weight management. Adv Nutr 1:17–30

Mehrabani HH, Salehpour S, Amiri Z et al (2012) Beneficial effects of a high-protein, low-glycemic-load hypocaloric diet in overweight and obese women with polycystic ovary syndrome: a randomized controlled intervention study. J Am Coll Nutr 31:117–125

Meyer KA, Kushi LH, Jacobs DR Jr et al (2000) Carbohydrates, dietary fiber, and incident type 2 diabetes in older women. Am J Clin Nutr 71:921–930

Miller V, Mente A, Dehghan M et al (2017) Fruit, vegetable, and legume intake, and cardiovascular disease and deaths in 18 countries (PURE): a prospective cohort study. Lancet 390:2037–2049

Mollard RC, Zykus A, Luhovyy BL et al (2012) The acute effects of a pulse-containing meal on glycaemic responses and measures of satiety and satiation within and at a later meal. Br J Nutr 108:509–517

Moran LJ, Hutchison SK, Norman RJ et al (2011) Lifestyle changes in women with polycystic ovary syndrome. Cochrane Database Syst Rev (7):Cd007506

Motta AB (2012) The role of obesity in the development of polycystic ovary syndrome. Curr Pharm Des 18:2482–2491. http://www.ingentaconnect.com/content/ben/cpd/2012/00000018/00000017/art00011. Accessed 27 Nov 2018

Mudryj AN, Yu N, Aukema HM (2014) Nutritional and health benefits of pulses. Appl Physiol Nutr Metab 39:1197–1204

Murtaugh MA, Sweeney C, Giuliano AR et al (2008) Diet patterns and breast cancer risk in Hispanic and non-Hispanic white women: the Four-Corners Breast Cancer Study. Am J Clin Nutr 87:978–984

National Cholesterol Education Program (NCEP) Expert Panel on Detection, Evaluation, and Treatment of High Blood Cholesterol in Adults (Adult Treatment Panel III) (2002) Third report of the National Cholesterol Education Program (NCEP) Expert Panel on Detection, Evaluation, and Treatment of High Blood Cholesterol in adults (Adult Treatment Panel III) final report. Circulation 106:3143–3421

Nestel P, Cehun M, Chronopoulos A (2004) Effects of long-term consumption and single meals of chickpeas on plasma glucose, insulin, and triacylglycerol concentrations. Am J Clin Nutr 79:390–395

Nnyepi M, Bennink MR, Jackson-Malete J et al (2015) Nutrition status of HIV+ children in Botswana. Health Educ 115:495–514

Noah L, Guillon F, Bouchet B et al (1998) Digestion of carbohydrate from white beans (*Phaseolus vulgaris* L.) in healthy humans. J Nutr 128:977–985

Odendo M, Bationo A, Kimani S (2011) Socio-economic contribution of legumes to livelihoods in Sub-Saharan Africa Fighting poverty in Sub-Saharan Africa: the multiple roles of legumes in Integrated Soil Fertility Management. Springer, Dordrecht, Netherlands, pp 27–46

Panizza CE, Shvetsov YB, Harmon BE et al (2018) Testing the predictive validity of the Healthy Eating Index-2015 in the multiethnic cohort: is the score associated with a reduced risk of all-cause and cause-specific mortality? Nutrients 10:452

Papanikolaou Y, Fulgoni VL III (2008) Bean consumption is associated with greater nutrient intake, reduced systolic blood pressure, lower body weight, and a smaller waist circumference in adults: results from the National Health and Nutrition Examination Survey 1999–2002. J Am Coll Nutr 27:569–576

Pilch SM (1987) Center for food safety and applied nutrition, federation of American societies for experimental biology and life sciences research office (contributors). Physiological effects and health consequences of dietary fiber. Bethesda, Maryland, United States, Life Sciences Research Office, Federation of American Societies for Experimental Biology

Reedy J, Lerman JL, Krebs-Smith SM et al (2018) Evaluation of the Healthy Eating Index-2015. J Acad Nutr Diet 118:1622–1633

Reverri EJ, Randolph JM, Kappagoda CT et al (2017) Assessing beans as a source of intrinsic fiber on satiety in men and women with metabolic syndrome. Appetite 118:75–81

Salas-Salvado J, Bullo M, Estruch R et al (2014) Prevention of diabetes with Mediterranean diets: a subgroup analysis of a randomized trial. Ann Intern Med 160:1–10

Schneeman BO (1987) Dietary fiber and gastrointestinal function. Nutr Rev 45:129–132

Shams H, Tahbaz F, Abadi A (2010) Effects of cooked lentils on glycemic control and blood lipids of patients with type 2 diabetes. ARYA Atheroscler 4(1):1–5

Sievenpiper JL, Kendall CW, Esfahani A et al (2009) Effect of non-oil-seed pulses on glycaemic control: a systematic review and meta-analysis of randomised controlled experimental trials in people with and without diabetes. Diabetologia 52:1479–1495

Souza RG, Gomes AC, Naves MM et al (2015) Nuts and legume seeds for cardiovascular risk reduction: scientific evidence and mechanisms of action. Nutr Rev 73:335–347

Stamets K, Taylor DS, Kunselman A et al (2004) A randomized trial of the effects of two types of short-term hypocaloric diets on weight loss in women with polycystic ovary syndrome. Fertil Steril 81:630–637

Teede HJ, Misso ML, Deeks AA et al (2011) Assessment and management of polycystic ovary syndrome: summary of an evidence-based guideline. Med J Aust 195:S65–S112

Teede HJ, Misso ML, Costello MF et al (2018) Recommendations from the international evidence-based guideline for the assessment and management of polycystic ovary syndrome. Hum Reprod 33:1602–1618

Thomson RL, Buckley JD, Noakes M et al (2008) The effect of a hypocaloric diet with and without exercise training on body composition, cardiometabolic risk profile, and reproductive function in overweight and obese women with polycystic ovary syndrome. J Clin Endocrinol Metab 93:3373–3380

Tielemans SM, Altorf-van Der Kuil W, Engberink MF et al (2013) Intake of total protein, plant protein and animal protein in relation to blood pressure: a meta-analysis of observational and intervention studies. J Hum Hypertens 27:564

Torsdottir I, Alpsten M, Andersson H et al (1989) Gastric emptying and glycemic response after ingestion of mashed bean or potato flakes in composite meals. Am J Clin Nutr 50:1415–1419

Tosh SM, Yada S (2010) Dietary fibres in pulse seeds and fractions: characterization, functional attributes, and applications. Food Res Int 43:450–460

Tovar J, Granfeldt Y, Bjoerck IM (1992) Effect of processing on blood glucose and insulin responses to starch in legumes. J Agric Food Chem 40:1846–1851

Tovar J, Nilsson A, Johansson M et al (2014) Combining functional features of whole-grain barley and legumes for dietary reduction of cardiometabolic risk: a randomised cross-over intervention in mature women. Br J Nutr 111:706–714

U.S. Department of Agriculture (USDA). Center for Nutrition and Policy Promotion. (2016) Inside the pyramid: how many vegetables are needed daily or weekly? http://fit4maui.com/pages/popUps/usda_veg.html. Accessed 27 Nov 2018

U.S. Department of Health and Human Services (USDHHS) (2017) Lower heart disease risk. https://www.nhlbi.nih.gov/health/educational/hearttruth/lower-risk/risk-factors.htm. Accessed 7 Dec 2018

U.S. Department of Health and Human Services (USDHHS) and U.S. Department of Agriculture (USDA) (n.d.) Dietary guidelines for Americans 2015–2020. http://health.gov/dietaryguidelines/2015/guidelines/. Accessed 7 Jul 2018

U.S. Food and Drug Administration (FDA) (2008) Guidance for industry diabetes mellitus: developing drugs and therapeutic biologics for treatment and prevention. https://www.fda.gov/downloads/Drugs/.../Guidances/ucm071624.pdf. Accessed 9 Dec 2018

Velie EM, Schairer C, Flood A et al (2005) Empirically derived dietary patterns and risk of postmenopausal breast cancer in a large prospective cohort study. Am J Clin Nutr 82:1308–1319

Venn B, Mann J (2004) Cereal grains, legumes and diabetes. Eur J Clin Nutr 58:1443–1461

Viguiliouk E, Blanco Mejia S, Kendall CW et al (2017) Can pulses play a role in improving cardiometabolic health? Evidence from systematic reviews and meta-analyses. Ann N Y Acad Sci 1392:43–57

Villegas R, Gao YT, Yang G et al (2008) Legume and soy food intake and the incidence of type 2 diabetes in the Shanghai Women's Health Study. Am J Clin Nutr 87:162–167

Wall CR, Stewart AW, Hancox RJ et al (2018) Association between frequency of consumption of fruit, vegetables, nuts and pulses and BMI: analyses of the International Study of Asthma and Allergies in Childhood (ISAAC). Nutrients 10:E316

Wang Y, Wang Z, Fu L et al (2013) Legume consumption and colorectal adenoma risk: a meta-analysis of observational studies. PLoS One 8:e67335

Wild RA, Carmina E, Diamanti-Kandarakis E et al (2010) Assessment of cardiovascular risk and prevention of cardiovascular disease in women with the polycystic ovary syndrome: a consensus statement by the Androgen Excess and Polycystic Ovary Syndrome (AE-PCOS) Society. J Clin Endocrinol Metab 95:2038–2049

Willig A, Wright L, Galvin TA (2018) Practice paper of the academy of nutrition and dietetics: nutrition intervention and human immunodeficiency virus infection. J Acad Nutr Diet 118:486–498

Wiseman M (2008) The second World Cancer Research Fund/American Institute for Cancer Research expert report. Food, nutrition, physical activity, and the prevention of cancer: a global perspective. Proc Nutr Soc 67:253–256

World Cancer Research Fund International (WCRF) (n.d.) Eat wholegrains, vegetables, fruit & beans. https://www.wcrf.org/dietandcancer/recommendations/wholegrains-veg-fruit-beans. Accessed 27 Nov 2018

Wright C, Zborowski J, Talbott E et al (2004) Dietary intake, physical activity, and obesity in women with polycystic ovary syndrome. Int J Obes Relat Metab Disord 28:1026–1032

Yao CK, Muir JG, Gibson PR (2016) Review article: insights into colonic protein fermentation, its modulation and potential health implications. Aliment Pharmacol Ther 43:181–196

Yildiz BO, Knochenhauer ES, Azziz R (2008) Impact of obesity on the risk for polycystic ovary syndrome. J Clin Endocrinol Metab 93:162–168

Zhu B, Sun Y, Qi L et al (2015) Dietary legume consumption reduces risk of colorectal cancer: evidence from a meta-analysis of cohort studies. Sci Rep 5:8797

# Chapter 6
# Pulses and Chronic Kidney Disease: Potential Health Benefits from a Once Forbidden Food

Fiona N. Byrne and Mona S. Calvo

**Abstract** Dietary treatment may slow the progression of chronic kidney disease (CKD), a condition where the ability to filter excess fluid and metabolic waste decreases over time. By restricting salt, protein, high phosphorus and potassium foods, better control over waste product and toxin build-up may be achieved in CKD. Hyperphosphatemia is a serious complication as CKD progresses since elevated serum phosphate can disrupt normal hormonal regulation of calcium and phosphorus leading to cardiovascular disease. Dietary restriction of phosphorus involves limiting high protein foods such as dairy, meat and some plant foods including pulses, largely due to their high phosphorus content. Restriction of pulses in renal diets have come into question since better health outcomes have been observed with diets higher in plant proteins. In this chapter, we reason that the high phosphorus content of pulses may not be sufficient to restrict a quality protein source such as pulses in renal diets since much of the phosphorus is not readily absorbed being bound-up in the form of phytate. We present evidence in support of the benefits of pulse consumption in CKD.

**Keywords** Pulses · Legumes · Chronic Kidney Disease · End Stage Renal Disease · Phosphorus · Calcium · Potassium · Plant protein · Dietary fiber · Acid-base balance · Phytate · Renal diet

F. N. Byrne
Department of Nutrition & Dietetics, Cork University Hospital, Cork, Ireland

Department of Nephrology, Cork University Hospital, Cork, Ireland

HRB Clinical Research Facility, University College Cork, Cork, Ireland
e-mail: fiona.byrne@hse.ie

M. S. Calvo (✉)
Retired, US Food and Drug Administration, Silver Spring, MD, USA
e-mail: mscalvo55@comcast.net

© Springer Nature Switzerland AG 2019
W. J. Dahl (ed.), *Health Benefits of Pulses*,
https://doi.org/10.1007/978-3-030-12763-3_6

## 6.1 Introduction

Chronic kidney disease (CKD) is a condition in which the kidneys are damaged or cannot filter blood as well as healthy kidneys. Because of this, excess fluid and waste from the blood remain in the body and may cause other health problems such as cardiovascular disease or metabolic bone disease. Kidney function usually gets worse over time, though dietary treatment may slow progression. When the kidneys stop working, dialysis or kidney transplant is needed for survival. Kidney failure treated with dialysis or kidney transplant is called end-stage renal disease (ESRD), but often CKD patients die before they reach this stage from cardiovascular disease complications (Centers for Disease Control and Prevention 2017). CKD is a common disease condition whose treatment is also expensive. For example, over 30 million people or 15% of United States (US) adults are estimated to have CKD. This equates to one in seven Americans. Medicare spending for all beneficiaries who had chronic kidney disease in 2015 (11% of total) exceeded $64 billion. When adding an extra $34 billion for ESRD costs, total Medicare spending on both CKD and ESRD was over $98 billion (US Renal Data System 2017).

The renal diet was developed with the intention of slowing the progression of the disease and to control the build-up of waste products. The renal diet introduces many dietary restrictions that become more burdensome depending on the stage of CKD (Table 6.1). In early CKD, patients are often advised to restrict salt. In moderate CKD, patients may be advised to restrict protein, which involves reducing dairy and other high animal protein foods such as meat. As CKD progresses and blood levels of potassium and phosphate rise, further dietary restrictions are introduced. The renal diet can be difficult to follow, restricting many common foods and can involve substantial change for patients that impact their quality of life.

Hyperphosphatemia or high blood phosphate is a common and serious complication that develops as CKD progresses. Treatment of hyperphosphatemia, focuses on

**Table 6.1** Recommended nutrient intakes according to CKD Stage (70 kg BW) (Kalantar-Zadeh and Fouque 2017)

| Nutrient | Mild-moderate CKD | Advanced CKD | Transition to dialysis |
|---|---|---|---|
| Protein[a] | 42–56 g/day | 42–56 g/day | 42–56 g/day |
| Phosphorus[b] | <800 mg/day | <800 mg/day | <800 mg/day |
| Sodium[c] | <4 g/day | <3 g/day | <3 g/day |
| Potassium | 4.7 g/day | <3 g/day | <3 g/day |
| Calcium[d] | 800–1000 mg/day | 800–1000 mg/day | 800–1000 mg/day or less |
| Fiber[e] | >25–30 g/day | >25–30 g/day | >25–30 g/day |

[a]Patients with advanced CKD should consume 50% high biological protein and 50% plant protein; better health outcomes have been observed in mild-moderate CKD patients who consumed diets with higher proportion of plant sources of protein (Chen et al. 2016)
[b]Minimize intake of highly processed foods containing phosphate food additives
[c]Minimize intake of highly processed foods
[d]Avoid foods that are fortified with calcium phosphate
[e]Consume higher proportion of minimally processed plant-based foods

dietary restriction of phosphorus in addition to the use of phosphorus binders to limit the amount of phosphorus that accumulates when the kidneys fail to excrete it in the urine. Elevated serum phosphate can trigger the disruption of the normal hormonal regulation of blood levels of phosphorus and calcium that can lead to soft tissue calcification, bone loss and cardiovascular disease (Haring et al. 2017; Kalantar-Zadeh and Fouque 2017). Phosphate binders are oral medications which bind dietary phosphorus in the gastrointestinal tract and can be used to prevent the absorption of a limited amount of dietary phosphorus. In ESRD, dialysis will also help to control phosphate levels, but it also has limitations with respect to phosphorous removal. As CKD progresses, potassium can also build up. Hyperkalaemia or high blood potassium is a serious complication that can also develop as CKD progresses and dietary restriction is an important means of controlling high blood potassium. Dietary restriction of phosphorus involves the restriction of high protein food particularly dairy products, avoidance of processed foods containing phosphate additives and avoidance of foods high in phosphorus such as cola, whole grains, chocolate, nuts and pulses (National Kidney Foundation 2017). Patients seeking dietary advice from the internet as to which foods to avoid to reduce their phosphorus and possibly potassium intakes will note that pulses such as lentils and dried beans are often listed as foods to avoid. Pulses are restricted on renal diets because of their high content of phosphorus and potassium. Table 6.2 presents examples from some frequently accessed websites that recommend pulses be limited or avoided when following a traditional renal diet.

Renal dietary restrictions have come under increased scrutiny in recent years with some questioning the effectiveness and evidence base which supports their use (Kalantar-Zadeh et al. 2015; Palmer et al. 2017). Better health outcomes have been observed in mild-moderate CKD patients who consumed diets with higher proportion of plant sources of protein (Chen et al. 2016; Haring et al. 2017; Moorthi and Moe 2018). Considering the growing health benefits of plant food consumption in CKD, nephrologists and renal dietitians are now calling into question the restriction of plant foods such as pulses that are sources of quality protein. High phosphorus content of pulses may not be reason enough to restrict their consumption if the phosphorus content of pulses is bound-up in the form of phytate, reducing phosphorus bioavailability (Byrne et al. 2017; Calvo et al. 2014). Pulse consumption contributes many other nutritional factors of potential benefit to renal patients. This chapter highlights the existing evidence in support of our speculation about the benefits of pulse consumption in CKD and aims for the safe and judicious inclusion of pulses in the renal diet.

## 6.2 The Challenge of the Renal Diet

When counseling patients about nutrition, renal dietitians aim to keep each patient well nourished, to ensure balance and incorporate healthy eating guidelines. Renal dietitians will also strive to integrate existing likes and dislikes and to maintain their

**Table 6.2** Current Internet websites providing dietary guidance for CKD/ESRD patients with selected examples of foods to avoid or limit when managing phosphorus intake

| Internet source | High phosphorus foods to avoid or limit |
|---|---|
| American Kidney Fund[a] | Dairy foods, *beans, lentils*, nuts, bran cereals, oatmeal, colas and other drinks with phosphate additives and some bottled ice teas |
| | Phosphate additives could add up to 1000 mg/day phosphorus; read the product label and look for phosphate or "phos" on the ingredient list |
| Mayo Clinic[b] | *Dried peas (split or black-eyed) beans (black, garbanzo, lima, kidney, navy, pinto) or lentils* |
| Cleveland Clinic[c] | "Some vegetables contain phosphorus, limit these to 1 cup/week: *dried beans…*" |
| | "Potassium-rich foods to avoid: *dried beans- -all kinds*" |
| National Kidney Disease Education Program[d] | *Beans (baked, kidney, lima, pinto)* |
| | Meat, poultry, fish, dairy foods, *beans, lentils,* nuts, bran cereals, oatmeal, colas, and some bottled ice teas |
| | Limit *beans and lentils* to ½ cup cooked |
| Familydoctor.org[e] | Dairy products (milk, cheese, yogurt and ice cream), *dried beans and peas (kidney beans, split peas, lentils)*, nuts and peanut butter, drinks like beer, cola, hot cocoa |
| DaVita – The Vegetarian Diet and Chronic Kidney Disease[f] | "Instead of *dried beans or peas*, have green beans or wax beans" |
| | "*Beans* and nuts are considered too high in potassium and phosphorus to be incorporated into a kidney diet. But with careful dietary planning with your dietitian, certain ones can be included in the vegetarian meal plan" |
| SFGATE[g] | "Because they are also rich in potassium, phosphorus, purines and oxalate, however, *lentils* are not an ideal choice for people affected by chronic kidney problems" |
| National Kidney Foundation[h] | "Ingredients to avoid: banana, cheese, chocolate, cocoa, coconut, cream, dried fruit, *dried peas and beans, lentils*" |

[a]Lauren Elkins (2015) Your kidney disease diet: Managing phosphorus. In: American Kidney Fund blog. Available at http://www.kidneyfund.org/kidney-today/your-kidney-disease-diet-managing-phosphorus.html. Accessed 27 Feb 2018

[b]Rachael Majorwicz (2012) Low-phosphorus diet: Best for kidney Disease. Why is a low-phosphorus diet useful in managing kidney disease? What foods contain phosphorus? In: Mayo Clinic blog. Available at http://www.mayoclinic.org/food.and.nutrition/expert.answers/faq-20058408. Accessed 27 Feb 2018

[c]Cleveland Clinic Renal Diet Basics. Available at http://www.my.clevelandclinic.org/health/articles/15641-renal-diet-basics. Accessed 27 Feb 2018

[d]National Kidney Disease Education Program High- and Low-phosphorus Foods. Available at https://www.niddk.nih.gov/health-information/kidney-disease/chronic-kidney-disease-ckd/eating-nutrition/nutrition-advanced-chronic-kidney-disease-adults Accessed 27 Feb 2018

[e]Familydoctor.org Nutrition for Advanced Chronic Kidney Disease in Adults. Available at https://familydoctor.org/chronic-kidney-disease-ckd-chronic-kidney-disease-nutrition/. Accessed 27 Feb 2018

[f]DaVita Phosphorus in Foods: What to know when you are on a kidney diet. Available at www.davita.com/kidney-disease/diet-and-nutrition/diet-basics/phosphorus-in-foods:-what-to-know-when-you're-on-a-kidney-diet/e/10253 The Vegetarian Diet and Chronic Kidney Disease https://www.davita.com/kidney-disease/diet-and-nutrition/lifestyle/the-vegetarian-diet-and-chronic-kidney-disease/e/5346. Accessed 27 Feb 2018.

[g]sfGate.com blog Are lentils harmful to kidneys? Available at http://healthyeating.sfgate.com/lentils-harmful-kidneys-12272.html. 24 Feb 2018.

[h]NKF: Your Guide to the New Food Label (2016). Available at https://www.kidney.org/atoz/content/foodlabel. Accessed 1 Feb 2018.

patient's enjoyment of food. Their ability to do this is, however, limited by the multiple nutrient restrictions such as protein, phosphate, sodium, and potassium, and the need to maintain adequate fiber intake, acid-base balance, and sufficient calcium intake, all factors that are critical to maintaining renal patient health.

## 6.3   Beneficial Aspects of Pulse Consumption to CKD Patients

### 6.3.1   Pulse Protein and Phosphorus Bioavailability

An important objective in dietary management of CKD is to aim for adequate protein intake while minimizing phosphorus intake. As shown in Fig. 6.1, there is a direct relationship between the phosphorus and protein content of diets (Byrne 2003). Because of the obligatory phosphorus load that comes with consuming high protein foods, it is difficult to restrict dietary phosphorus. However some foods contain more phosphorus per gram of protein than others. This has led some experts to focus on the phosphorus to protein ratio, also expressed as mg phosphorus/g protein. Significant links have been established between high phosphorus to protein ratios and incident mortality (Noori et al. 2010). Animal protein such as meat and

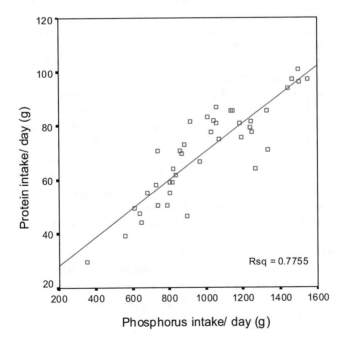

**Fig. 6.1**  Relationship between protein and phosphorus intakes (Byrne 2003)

chicken provide approximately 7–12 mg phosphorus/g protein (Kalantar-Zadeh 2013) whereas pulses have a much higher apparent ratio (Table 6.3).When we consider bioavailability and lower absorption rates due to the phytate content, pulses become more comparable to animal proteins with respect to the phosphorus/protein ratio (Barril-Cuadrado et al. 2013).

The *Phosphorus Pyramid* (shown in text form in Fig. 6.2) was designed to be used as a visual tool for CKD/ESRD patients to use for management of phosphorus intake. In designing the pyramid, the authors used the phosphorus/protein ratio to identify foods with favourable phosphorus to protein content, setting an upper limit of 12 mg phosphorus/g protein. Two other factors were used for placement of foods at one of the six pyramid levels. These were bioavailability of phosphorus and the presence of phosphate additives, both of which influence the actual phosphorus load (Cupisti and Kalantar-Zadeh 2013; D'Alessandro et al. 2015). The *Phosphorus Pyramid*, similar to that first introduced in the USA by the Department of Agriculture in 1992, graphically shows the recommended frequency (daily, weekly or less) and the relative amount of specific food groups to consume based on its position and size of the section in the pyramid (D'Alessandro et al. 2015). The foods on the bottom of the pyramid should be consumed most frequently whilst those at the top should be consumed least frequently.

On first inspection, the high phosphorus/protein ratio of the pulses shown in Table 6.3 suggests that they are unsuitable for inclusion in CKD diets. However, these pulses also contain high levels of phytate, the dominant form of phosphorus in plant-based protein. While the phosphorus content is high in pulses, the presence of phytate has been shown to significantly slow the rate and efficiency of phosphorus absorption resulting in very low phosphorus bioavailability from plant-based proteins (Itkonen et al. 2012, 2018; Itkonen and Lamberg-Allardt 2017; Karp et al. 2012). Dietary phosphorus is absorbed from three basic food sources: animal protein (organic), plant protein (organic) and phosphorus additives (inorganic) used in food processing. Each source differs in their phosphorus bioavailability (Calvo and Uribarri 2013; Kalantar-Zadeh et al. 2010). Experts consider phosphorus food additives to be the most efficiently and rapidly absorbed (80–100%), followed by animal protein with absorption rates of 60–80% and plant protein bioavailability at only 20–40%. Specific to pulses, despite their relatively high total phosphorus content, they are poor sources of bioavailable phosphorus showing 6–42% absorption in in vitro digestion models that mimic the human gut and digestion process (Itkonen et al. 2012; Karp et al. 2012). The phytate content of pulses is about 30% or more of total pulse phosphorus content which justifies recalculating the phosphorus to protein ratio (Barril-Cuadrado et al. 2013; Davies and Warrington 1986; Egli et al. 2002; Lukmanji et al. 2008; Oatway et al. 2001). Using a 40% bioavailability of phosphorus and adjusting for poor bioavailability determined more favourable phosphorus/protein ratios and explains why pulses are included in the second shelf of the pyramid, below all the animal proteins despite their apparent higher phosphorus/protein ratio (D'Alessandro et al. 2015).

**Table 6.3** Nutrient content and estimated phosphorus/protein ratio with/without adjustment for phytate content

| Pulse[c] | Protein | Carbohydrate | Fiber | Phosphorus | Calcium | Sodium | Potassium | Apparent mg P/g protein | Phytate adjusted[a] | Phytate[b] |
|---|---|---|---|---|---|---|---|---|---|---|
| | g/100 g | | | mg/100 g | | | | | mg P/g protein | g/100 g dry weight |
| Adzuki beans | 7.5 | 24.8 | 7.3 | 168 | 28 | 8 | 532 | 22.4 | 8.9 | ~ |
| Small white beans | 8.97 | 25.81 | 10.4 | 169 | 73 | 2 | 463 | 18.8 | 7.6 | 1.13[b1] |
| Great Northern beans | 8.33 | 21.09 | 7.0 | 165 | 68 | 2 | 391 | 19.8 | 7.9 | 1.12[b3] |
| Pink beans | 9.06 | 27.91 | 5.3 | 165 | 52 | 2 | 508 | 18.2 | 7.3 | ~ |
| Black beans | 8.86 | 23.71 | 8.7 | 140 | 27 | 1 | 355 | 15.8 | 6.3 | 0.86[b1] |
| Black turtle beans | 8.18 | 24.35 | 8.3 | 152 | 55 | 3 | 433 | 18.6 | 7.4 | ~ |
| Lentils | 9.02 | 20.13 | 7.9 | 180 | 19 | 2 | 369 | 20.0 | 8.0 | 1.15[b1] 0.36[d, b2] |
| Pinto beans | 9.01 | 26.22 | 5.3 | 147 | 46 | 1 | 436 | 16.3 | 6.5 | 0.93[b3] |
| Kidney beans | 9.13 | 22.41 | 9.3 | 137 | 66 | 4 | 419 | 15.3 | 6.02 | 1.59[b2] 0.62[d, b2] |
| Navy beans | 8.23 | 26.05 | 10.5 | 144 | 69 | 0 | 389 | 17.5 | 7.0 | 1.09[b3] |
| Cow peas[h] | 7.73 | 20.76 | 6.5 | 156 | 24 | 4 | 278 | 20.2 | 8.0 | 0.94[b2] 0.66[d, b1] |
| Lima beans | 7.80 | 20.88 | 7.0 | 111 | 17 | 2 | 508 | 14.2 | 5.6 | 0.84[b3] |
| Chickpeas[i] | 8.86 | 27.42 | 7.6 | 168 | 49 | 7 | 291 | 19.0 | 7.6 | 0.48[b1] |
| Pigeon peas | 6.76 | 23.25 | 6.7 | 119 | 43 | 5 | 385 | 17.6 | 7.0 | 1.15[b2] 0.40[d, b2] |
| Cranberry beans[j] | 9.34 | 24.46 | 8.6 | 135 | 50 | 1 | 387 | 14.4 | 5.8 | ~ |
| Split peas | 8.34 | 21.10 | 8.3 | 99 | 14 | 2 | 362 | 11.9 | 4.8 | 0.63[b1] |

(continued)

**Table 6.3** (continued)

| | Protein | Carbohydrate | Fiber | Phosphorus | Calcium | Sodium | Potassium | Apparent mg P/g protein | Phytate adjusted[a] | Phytate[b] |
|---|---|---|---|---|---|---|---|---|---|---|
| Pulse[c] | g/100 g | | | mg/100 g | | | | | mg P/g protein | g/100 g dry weight |
| Mung beans | 7.02 | 19.15 | 7.06 | 99 | 27 | 2 | 266 | 14.10 | 5.7 | 0.945[b2] |
| | | | | | | | | | | 0.11[d] |

[a]P/Protein ratio adjusted for phytate content was estimated using a reduced phosphorus value conservatively based on a 40% absorption efficiency (Itkonen and Lamberg-Allardt (2017). *Apparent* P/protein ratio was calculated by dividing the phosphorus content in 100 g by the protein content in 100 g (mg/g)

[b]Data source for Phytate content: values indicated with [b1]from Egli et al. (2002); values indicated [b2]from Lukmanji et al. (2008) and values indicated [b3]from Oatway et al. (2001). Unless otherwise indicated, all phytate content is for dry weight of raw or uncooked pulses

[c]Nutrient content of pulses from USDA Nutrient Database for Standard Reference Release 28, slightly revised May 2016. Data report January 23, 2018. All pulses were cooked, boiled without salt

[d]Indicates phytate content of cooked pulse rather than uncooked or raw

[e]Cow peas, also known as black eyes, crowder and southern peas

[f]Chickpeas, also known as Garbanzo beans, Bengal gram

[g]Cranberry beans also known as Romano beans

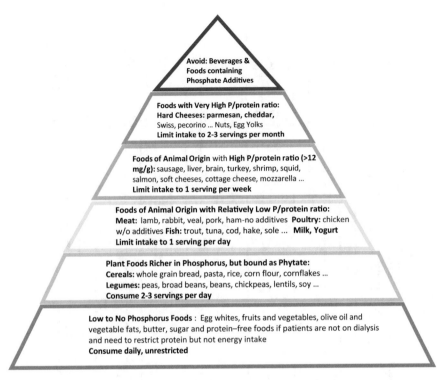

**Fig. 6.2** Modified Text version of the *Phosphorus Pyramid* (Adapted from D'Alessandro et al. 2015)

### 6.3.2   Pulse as a Source of Quality Protein

There are two parts to assessing protein quality. The first consideration looks at the amino acid profile and the second at the digestibility. It is well known that the concentration of certain indispensable amino acids is lower in plant-based proteins than in animal proteins and in general, plant proteins are of lower biological value than animal proteins that contain sufficient levels of all the essential amino acids (Institute of Medicine 2005; Young and Pellett 1994). Table 6.4 reports the amino acid profiles of commonly consumed pulses compared to the 2007 WHO indispensable amino acid requirements for adults (Joint WHO/FAO/UNU Expert Consultation 2007). On inspection, pulses do not appear to be lacking in indispensable amino acids relative to the adult requirement, except for kidney beans that are low in aromatic amino acids and chickpeas low in aromatic and sulphur amino acids. The second part looks at digestibility of the protein source. In general, protein in cooked pulses is highly digestible (Nosworthy et al. 2017).

In the United States, protein quality is evaluated by the PDCAAS (Protein Digestibility Corrected Amino Acid Score) that combines measures of both the digestibility and amino acid score into a score between 0 and 1. Under U.S. labelling

**Table 6.4** Protein quality evaluation of pulses (WHO/FAO/UNU 2007)

| | Histidine | Isoleucine | Leucine | Lysine | Methionine + Cystine | Phenyl-alanine + Tyrosine | Threonine | Tryptophan | Valine | Total minus histidine |
|---|---|---|---|---|---|---|---|---|---|---|
| Estimated essential amino acid requirements | | | | | | | | | | |
| mg/g protein | | | | | | | | | | |
| Adults ≥18 years | 15 | 30 | 59 | 45 | 22 | 30 | 23 | 6 | 39 | 254 |
| Pulse | Essential amino acid profile of commonly consumed pulses[a] | | | | | | | | | |
| | mg/g protein | | | | | | | | | |
| Lentils | 28 | 43 | 72 | 70 | 22 | 63 | 36 | 9 | 50 | 333 |
| Chickpeas | 28 | 43 | 71 | 67 | 15 | 22 | 37 | 10 | 42 | 323 |
| Kidney beans | 28 | 44 | 80 | 69 | 26 | 19 | 42 | 12 | 52 | 407 |
| Cowpeas | 26 | 40 | 76 | 68 | 25 | 76 | 38 | 12 | 48 | 399 |
| Black beans | 28 | 44 | 80 | 69 | 26 | 78 | 42 | 12 | 68 | 343 |
| Pinto beans | 13 | 51 | 85 | 70 | 22 | 82 | 36 | 12 | 58 | 416 |
| Navy beans | 25 | 47 | 85 | 63 | 23 | 81 | 35 | 12 | 61 | 407 |
| Lima beans | 31 | 53 | 86 | 67 | 24 | 93 | 43 | 12 | 60 | 438 |
| Pigeon peas | 31 | 37 | 72 | 71 | 22 | 110 | 35 | 10 | 43 | 400 |
| Split-peas | 24 | 41 | 72 | 72 | 25 | 75 | 35 | 11 | 47 | 378 |
| Cranberry beans | 28 | 44 | 81 | 69 | 26 | 82 | 42 | 12 | 52 | 408 |
| Pink beans | 28 | 44 | 80 | 69 | 26 | 82 | 42 | 12 | 52 | 407 |
| Mung beans | 26 | 38 | 77 | 70 | 21 | 89 | 33 | 11 | 51 | 390 |
| Soybeans[b] | 25 | 44 | 74 | 61 | 27 | 82 | 40 | 13 | 46 | 387 |

[a] Amino acid content of the pulses was estimated from the mg amino acid content in 100 g of pulse divided by the protein content in 100 g of the pulse to yield mg amino acid/g pulse protein. All amino acid and protein data were provided by USDA Nutrient Database for Standard Release 28, slightly revised May 2016, Accessed 23 Jan 2018
[b] Reference food

regulations for adult foods, a protein must have a PDCAAS value greater than 0.2 (20%) to qualify as a quality protein (Food and Drug Administration 2017). As shown in Table 6.5, pulses have a PDCAAS score of 0.5 or greater (Nosworthy et al. 2017). A newly accepted alternative way to evaluate protein quality based on indispensable amino acid composition and digestibility is the DIAAS score (Digestible Indispensable Amino Acid Score) (FAO/WHO 2013) and values for cooked Canadian pulses are shown in Table 6.5. In the European Union, pulses providing greater than 20% of the energy as protein qualify as "High in Protein" (European Union 2006). Pulse protein biological value may not be comparable with many animal proteins, but pulses are among the highest quality plant proteins such as soy.

There is increasing interest in sarcopenia (loss of muscle), a condition detrimental to our renal patients and aging population. Protein quality, dose and timing, as well as exercise, are all factors which may affect muscle synthesis, loss of strength and impact bone in CKD. With respect to muscle degradation and synthesis, an adequate intake of the indispensable amino acid leucine is critical (Phillips 2016).

**Table 6.5** Protein quality of cooked Canadian pulses using the United States regulatory standards for protein evaluation (Nosworthy et al. 2017)

| Pulse | Protein, cooked | PDCAAS[a] | Corrected protein per serving | % daily value[b] | DIAAS[c] | Qualify for a good source of protein claim in US[d] |
|---|---|---|---|---|---|---|
| | g/100 g | – | 90 g | 50 g | – | – |
| Red kidney beans | 8.27 | 0.549 | 4.09 | 8.17 | 0.51 | Yes |
| Navy beans | 8.76 | 0.667 | 5.26 | 10.52 | 0.65 | Yes |
| Whole green lentils | 6.72 | 0.628 | 3.80 | 7.60 | 0.58 | – |
| Split red lentils | 7.30 | 0.538 | 3.54 | 7.07 | 0.50 | – |
| Split yellow peas | 6.81 | 0.643 | 3.94 | 7.87 | 0.73 | Yes |
| Split green peas | 7.39 | 0.500 | 3.33 | 6.65 | 0.46 | – |
| Black beans | 8.39 | 0.534 | 4.03 | 8.07 | 0.49 | Yes |
| Chickpeas | 7.57 | 0.519 | 3.53 | 7.07 | 0.67 | Yes |
| Pinto beans | 7.85 | 0.590 | 4.17 | 8.33 | 0.60 | Yes |

[a]PDCAAS is the Protein Digestibility-Corrected Amino Acid Score used in the United Stated to evaluate protein quality. In the US, for adults and children over 4 years, to qualify as a quality protein, the protein source must have a PDCAAS score greater than 0.2 (20%)
[b]% Daily value is the reference amount of daily protein intake used on the FDA Nutrient Facts label to let consumers track the adequacy of their protein intake. The Daily Value for protein is 50 g and the protein content of the food is usually expressed as a percent of this value or in g/serving
[c]Digestible Indispensable Amino Acid Score (DIAAS) values determination first considers protein digestibility followed by the value of the first limiting amino acid. Note, no country or regulatory group has set this method in use yet, but it is more accurate in terms of estimating protein quality
[d]In the U.S., specific to foods for adults and children over 4 years, to qualify as a good source of protein, the protein food must have a PDCAAS score greater than 0.2 (20%)

Leucine and other branch chain amino acids are notably rich in pulses and may serve as an important source in the early stages of CKD where low serum concentrations of leucine have been reported (Kumar et al. 2012). The benefits of pulses to sarcopenia in CKD need further study since van Vliet et al. provided evidence that some plant proteins produce a lower muscle protein synthetic response compared to animal-based proteins (van Vliet et al. 2015). Plant sources of protein may need to be combined with animal or other plant proteins to ensure a complete balanced amino acid bolus is delivered to the muscle to maximize muscle protein synthesis.

### 6.3.3   Pulses, Phosphorus, Sodium and Potassium

Phosphorus, potassium, and sodium are all nutrients of interest in CKD/ESKD. Pulses are naturally rich in protein, phosphorus, and potassium and low in sodium. Table 6.6 compares the composition of pulses prepared in different ways and demonstrates the effect that cooking methods can have on the nutrient profiles of pulses. To the benefit of renal patients, the protein content of pulses remains largely unchanged regardless of the cooking method, while the mineral content can change.

The significant phosphorus content of pulses is largely phytate bound which reduces its bioavailability (Schlemmer et al. 2009). We have argued that their higher phosphorus content is therefore not a cause for concern and the method of cooking pulses can further reduce their phosphorus content. The phosphorus content of canned pulses is lower than home cooked pulses as shown in Table 6.6. Pulses are rich in potassium and this may be a concern if blood potassium levels are elevated. Canned pulses are lower in potassium than home cooked pulses and so may be a better choice. Canned pulses in water (without added salt) are the most suitable for CKD patients as they are lower in phosphorus and potassium than home cooked pulses and they are low in sodium (Table 6.6).

### 6.3.4   Pulses and Dietary Fiber

Fiber has an important role in the health and wellbeing of humans (Dahl and Stewart 2015). In CKD, there is a dysbiosis or imbalance of the intestinal microflora (Evenepoel et al. 2009; Guldris et al. 2017) and this has adverse effects on the immune system (Anders et al. 2013) and may lead to inflammation (Lau et al. 2015). Fiber may improve gastrointestinal dysbiosis in two ways. First, fermentable fibers yield short chain fatty acids (SCFA) which provides energy to the mucosal wall, maintaining integrity. Second, fermentation provides energy to the intestinal flora and allows proteins and amino acids that reach the colon to be incorporated into bacterial proteins and be excreted instead of fermented into uremic solutes (Guldris et al. 2017). The inclusion of amino acids, into bacterial protein, may prevent the build-up of uremic toxins such as *p*-cresyl sulfate (PCS) (Meijers et al. 2010;

**Table 6.6** Evidence of cooking/canning change in sodium, potassium and phosphorus content, and protein and fiber content of commonly eaten pulses

| Prepared Pulse | Protein | Fiber | Sodium | Potassium | Phosphorus |
|---|---|---|---|---|---|
| | mg/100 g | | | | |
| Chickpeas[a] *drained* (home cooked v canned rinsed) | | | | | |
| Chickpeas mature seeds cooked boiled w/o salt | 8.9 | 7.6 | 7 | 291 | 168 |
| Chickpeas mature seeds canned drained solids | 7.1 | 6.4 | 246 | 126 | 85 |
| Chickpeas mature seeds canned drained rinsed in tap water | 7 | 6.3 | 212 | 109 | 80 |
| Chickpeas canned | | | | | |
| Chickpeas mature seeds canned solids and liquids | 4.9 | 4.4 | 278 | 144 | 80 |
| Chickpeas mature seeds canned solids and liquids low sodium | 4.9 | 4.4 | 132 | 144 | 80 |
| Kidney Beans *drained* (home cooked v canned v canned rinsed) | | | | | |
| Beans Kidney all types mature seeds cooked boiled w/o salt | 8.7 | 6.4 | 1 | 405 | 138 |
| Beans Kidney red mature canned drained solids | 8 | 5.5 | 231 | 277 | 121 |
| Beans Kidney red mature seeds canned drained solids rinsed in tap water | 8.1 | 6 | 208 | 250 | 118 |
| Kidney Beans *canned* | | | | | |
| Beans Kidney red mature seeds canned solids and liquids | 5.2 | 4.3 | 256 | 260 | 106 |
| Beans Kidney red mature seeds canned solids and liquid low sodium | 5.2 | 5.3 | 117 | 260 | 106 |
| Chicken (reference food) mg/25 g chicken | | | | | |
| Chicken broiler or fryers breast skinless boneless meat only cooked grilled | 7.6 | 0 | 13 | 98 | 65 |

Nutrient content of prepared pulses from USDA Nutrient Database for Standard Reference Release 28, slightly revised May 2016. Data report January 23, 2018
[a]Chickpeas are also known as Garbanzo beans or Bengal gram

Salmean et al. 2015) and indoxyl sulfate (IS) (Sirich et al. 2014). When compared to non-vegetarians, vegetarians with CKD have lower levels of these uremic toxins (Kandouz et al. 2016; Patel et al. 2012). These uremic toxins are harmful as they may trigger vascular inflammation and subsequently induce a systemic inflammatory response (Evenepoel and Meijers 2012). They have also been shown to have a role in vascular and renal disease progression (Vanholder et al. 2014). An increase in fiber intake has also been associated with reduced inflammation and reduced mortality in CKD populations (Krishnamurthy et al. 2012). While this research is promising it is not conclusive. Pulse consumption has been shown to be beneficial in the prevention of chronic disease in non CKD populations (Ha et al. 2014; Micha et al. 2017; Viguiliouk et al. 2017). Pulse consumption is associated with a lower risk of CKD (Haring et al. 2017) although Liu et al. (2017) were only able to show this effect in subjects with hypertension. Pulse consumption is also associated with a slowing of progression of CKD (Gluba-Brzozka et al. 2017). These findings merit further study of pulse consumption in this vulnerable population to determine the beneficial nutrient components of pulses.

### 6.3.5 Pulses and Maintenance of Acid-Base Balance

Metabolic acidosis (low serum bicarbonate) occurs frequently in CKD and is caused by the damaged kidney's inability to excrete acid. Metabolic acidosis has been associated with bone disease, muscle dysfunction, and kidney damage. Correction of acidosis through supplementation of sodium bicarbonate has been shown to slow progression of CKD and to improve nutritional status (de Brito-Ashurst et al. 2009). Consumption of a higher percentage of protein from plant sources may also raise bicarbonate (Scialla et al. 2012). In a related area of research, efforts to reduce acid load through the inclusion of fruit and vegetables have shown promise in delaying the progression of CKD (Goraya et al. 2013, 2014). Partial replacement of animal protein with some pulses may reduce the dietary acid load, and thus may be beneficial to patients with CKD.

## 6.4 Limitations to the Use of Pulses in CKD

The high phytate content of pulses is considered by some an antinutrient which may reduce absorption of other minerals such as calcium, zinc, and iron (Schlemmer et al. 2009). The renal diet traditionally restricts dairy and consequently calcium to achieve phosphate restriction, however calcium intakes were often supplemented with the use of calcium-based phosphate binders (Byrne et al. 2009). Recent Kidney Disease Improving Global Outcomes (KDIGO) guidelines suggest restricting calcium-based binders (Kidney Disease Improving Global Outcomes (KDIGO) CKD-MBD Update Work Group 2017) and their use is declining (St Peter et al. 2018). In the future, we may need to pay more attention to the calcium content of renal diets and specifically the calcium to phosphorus ratio as this may be of concern in terms of optimizing bone health in CKD patients. This will be particularly important if we are going to advise an increase in pulse consumption as phytates may reduce absorption of minerals such as calcium (Schlemmer et al. 2009).

A second limitation is that pulses are naturally high in potassium and a high blood potassium is a serious complication that can occur as CKD becomes more advanced either as a result of reduced kidney function or through the use of important medications such as angiotensin-converting-enzyme inhibitors (ACEs). Until we have further safety evidence, caution needs to be exercised in patients who have high blood potassium levels.

## 6.5 Future Use of Pulses in Renal Diets

Patients with CKD or ESKD should talk to a registered dietitian before changing their diet. It may be possible to safely replace some of the animal protein in the diets of patients with CKD and ESKD with more plant protein, such as pulses. Pulses provide quality protein and extra fiber, they are cheap and sustainable, and they add variety to a limited diet. Research is underway to provide valuable information on the efficacy, safety and tolerability of a modified renal diet, including plant protein sources such as pulses (Byrne et al. 2018).

## References

Anders H-J, Andersen K, Stecher B (2013) The intestinal microbiota, a leaky gut, and abnormal immunity in kidney disease. Kidney Int 83:1010–1016

Barril-Cuadrado G, Puchulu MB, Sanchez-Tomero JA (2013) Table showing dietary phosphorus/protein ratio for the Spanish population. Usefulness in chronic kidney disease. Nefrologia 33:362–371. https://doi.org/10.3265/Nefrologia.pre2013.Feb.11918

de Brito-Ashurst I, Varagunam M et al (2009) Bicarbonate supplementation slows progression of CKD and improves nutritional status. J Am Soc Nephrol 20:2075–2084

Byrne FN (2003) The effect of eating patterns on nutritional status and phosphate control in haemodialysis patients. Masters Thesis, The National University of Ireland Cork

Byrne FN, Kinsella S, Murnaghan DJ et al (2009) Lack of correlation between calcium intake and serum calcium levels in stable haemodialysis subjects. Nephron Clin Pract 113:c162–c168

Byrne F, Gillman B, Gleeson B et al (2017) Comparison of two diets with different phosphorus contents and bioavailability on serum phosphate levels in haemodialysis patients. Nephrol Dial Transplant 32(suppl 3):iii683–iii683

Byrne FN, Eustace, J, Gillman, BA (2018) Multicentre randomized control trial of phosphate control with a modified as compared to standard renal diet. Paper presented at Kidney Week 2018, San Diego, 25 October 2018

Calvo MS, Uribarri J (2013) Contributions to total phosphorus intake: all sources considered. Semin Dial 26:54–61. https://doi.org/10.1111/sdi.12042

Calvo MS, Moshfegh AJ, Tucker KL (2014) Assessing the health impact of phosphorus in the food supply: issues and considerations. Adv Nutr 5:104–113

Center for Diease Control and Prevention (2017) National chronic kidney disease fact sheet. Published by the Centers for Diease Control and Prevention, US Department of Health and Human Services, Atlanta, GA

Chen X, Wei G, Jalili T et al (2016) The associations of plant protein intake with all-cause mortality in CKD. Am J Kidney Dis 67:423–430

Cupisti A, Kalantar-Zadeh K (2013) Management of natural and added dietary phosphorus burden in kidney disease. Semin Nephrol 33:180–190

D'Alessandro C, Piccoli GB, Cupisti A (2015) The "phosphorus pyramid": a visual tool for dietary phosphate management in dialysis and CKD patients. BMC Nephrol 16:1–6

Dahl WJ, Stewart ML (2015) Position of the Academy of Nutrition and Dietetics: health implications of dietary fiber. J Acad Nutr Diet 115:1861–1870

Davies NT, Warrington S (1986) The phytic acid mineral, trace element, protein and moisture content of UK Asian immigrant foods. Hum Nutr Appl Nutr 40:49–59

Egli I, Davidsson L, Juillerat MA et al (2002) The influence of soaking and germination on the phytase activity and phytic acid content of grains and seeds potentially useful for complementary feeding. J Food Sci 67:3484–3488

Evenepoel P, Meijers BK (2012) Dietary fiber and protein: nutritional therapy in chronic kidney disease and beyond. Kidney Int 81:227–229

Evenepoel P, Meijers BK, Bammens BR et al (2009) Uremic toxins originating from colonic microbial metabolism. Kidney Int Suppl 76(114):S12–S19. https://doi.org/10.1038/ki.2009.402

FAO/WHO (2013) Dietary protein quality evaluation in human nutrition. Report of an FAO Expert Consultation. http://www.fao.org/ag/humannutrition/35978-02317b979a686a57aa4593304f-fc17f06.pdf. Accessed 23 Nov 2018

Food and Drug Administration (2017) Food labeling: revision of the nutrition and supplements facts labels. (FDA-2012-N-1210). Federal Register

Gluba-Brzozka A, Franczyk B, Rysz J (2017) Vegetarian diet in chronic kidney disease-a friend or foe. Nutrients 9:374. https://doi.org/10.3390/nu9040374

Goraya N, Simoni J, Jo C-H et al (2013) A comparison of treating metabolic acidosis in CKD stage 4 hypertensive kidney disease with fruits and vegetables or sodium bicarbonate. Clin J Am Soc Nephrol 8:371–381

Goraya N, Simoni J, Jo CH et al (2014) Treatment of metabolic acidosis in patients with stage 3 chronic kidney disease with fruits and vegetables or oral bicarbonate reduces urine angiotensinogen and preserves glomerular filtration rate. Kidney Int 86:1031–1038

Guldris SC, Parra EG, Amenós AC (2017) Gut microbiota in chronic kidney disease. Nefrología (English Edition) 37:9–19

Ha V, Sievenpiper JL, de Souza RJ et al (2014) Effect of dietary pulse intake on established therapeutic lipid targets for cardiovascular risk reduction: a systematic review and meta-analysis of randomized controlled trials. CMAJ 186:E252–E262

Haring B, Selvin E, Liang M et al (2017) Dietary protein sources and risk for incident chronic kidney disease: results from the Atherosclerosis Risk in Communities (ARIC) study. J Ren Nutr 27:233–242

Institute of Medicine (2005) Dietary reference intakes for energy, carbohydrate, fiber, fat, fatty acids, cholesterol, protein, and amino acids. The National Academies Press, Washington, D.C.

Itkonen ST, Lamberg-Allardt CJE (2017) Letter to the editor re: McClure et al. nutrients 2017, 9, 95. Nutrients 9:585

Itkonen ST, Ekholm PJ, Kemi VE et al (2012) Analysis of in vitro digestible phosphorus content in selected processed rye, wheat and barley products. J Food Compos Anal 25:185–189

Itkonen S, Karp H, Lamberg-Allardt C (2018) Bioavailability of phosphorus. In: Uribarri J, Calvo MS (eds) Dietary phosphorus health, nutrition and regulatory aspects. CRC Press, Boca Raton, pp 221–233

Joint WHO/FAO/UNU Expert Consultation (2007) Protein and amino acid requirements in human nutrition. WHO Technical Report Series 935. http://apps.who.int/iris/handle/10665/43411. Accessed 23 Nov 2018

Kalantar-Zadeh K (2013) Patient education for phosphorus management in chronic kidney disease. Patient Prefer Adherence 7:379–390

Kalantar-Zadeh K, Fouque D (2017) Nutritional management of chronic kidney disease. N Engl J Med 377:1765–1776

Kalantar-Zadeh K, Gutekunst L, Mehrotra R et al (2010) Understanding sources of dietary phosphorus in the treatment of patients with chronic kidney disease. Clin J Am Soc Nephrol 5:519–530

Kalantar-Zadeh K, Tortorici AR, Chen JLT et al (2015) Dietary restrictions in dialysis patients: is there anything left to eat? Semin Dial 28:159–168

Kandouz S, Mohamed AS, Zheng Y et al (2016) Reduced protein bound uraemic toxins in vegetarian kidney failure patients treated by haemodiafiltration. Hemodial Int 20:610–617

Karp H, Ekholm P, Kemi V et al (2012) Differences among total and in vitro digestible phosphorus content of meat and milk products. J Ren Nutr 22:344–349

Kidney Disease Improving Global Outcomes (KDIGO) CKD-MBD Update Work Group (2017) KDIGO 2017 clinical practice guideline update for the diagnosis, evaluation, prevention, and treatment of Chronic Kidney Disease–Mineral and Bone Disorder (CKD-MBD). Kidney Int Suppl 7:1–59

Krishnamurthy VM, Wei G, Baird BC et al (2012) High dietary fiber intake is associated with decreased inflammation and all-cause mortality in patients with chronic kidney disease. Kidney Int 81:300–306

Kumar MA, Bitla AR, Raju KV et al (2012) Branched chain amino acid profile in early chronic kidney disease. Saudi J Kidney Dis Transpl 23:1202–1207

Lau WL, Kalantar-Zadeh K, Vaziri ND (2015) The gut as a source of inflammation in chronic kidney disease. Nephron 130:92–98

Liu Y, Kuczmarski MF, Miller ER et al (2017) Dietary habits and risk of kidney function decline in an urban population. J Ren Nutr 27:16–25

Lukmanji Z, Hertmark E, Mlingi N et al (2008) Tanzania food composition tables, 1st edn. Muhimbili University College of Health and Allied Sciences and Tanzania Food and Nutrition Center, Dar es Salaam, Tanzania and Harvard School of Public Health, Boston

Meijers BK, De Preter V, Verbeke K et al (2010) p-Cresyl sulfate serum concentrations in hae-modialysis patients are reduced by the prebiotic oligofructose-enriched inulin. Nephrol Dial Transplant 25:219–224

Micha R, Shulkin ML, Peñalvo JL et al (2017) Etiologic effects and optimal intakes of foods and nutrients for risk of cardiovascular diseases and diabetes: systematic reviews and meta-analyses from the Nutrition and Chronic Diseases Expert Group (NutriCoDE). PLoS One 12:e0175149. https://doi.org/10.1371/journal.pone.0175149

Moorthi RN, Moe SM (2018) Special nutritional needs of chronic kidney and end-stage renal disease patients: rationale for the use of plant-based diets. In: Uribarri J, Calvo MS (eds) Dietary phosphorus, health, nutrition and regulatory aspects. CRC Press, Boca Raton, pp 235–246

National Kidney Foundation (2017) If you need to limit phosphorus. https://www.kidney.org/sites/default/files/02-10-0411_ABB_Phosphorus.pdf. Accessed 23 Nov 2018

Noori N, Kalantar-Zadeh K, Kovesdy CP et al (2010) Association of dietary phosphorus intake and phosphorus to protein ratio with mortality in hemodialysis patients. Clin J Am Soc Nephrol 5:683–692

Nosworthy MG, Neufeld J, Frohlich P et al (2017) Determination of the protein quality of cooked Canadian pulses. Food Sci Nutr 5:896–903

Oatway L, Vasanthan T, Helm JH (2001) Phytic acid. Food Rev Int 17:419–431

Palmer SC, Maggo JK, Campbell KL et al (2017) Dietary interventions for adults with chronic kidney disease. Cochrane Database Syst Rev 4:CD011998. https://doi.org/10.1002/14651858.CD011998.pub2

Patel KP, Luo FJ, Plummer NS et al (2012) The production of p-cresol sulfate and indoxyl sulfate in vegetarians versus omnivores. Clin J Am Soc Nephrol 7:982–988

Phillips SM (2016) The impact of protein quality on the promotion of resistance exercise-induced changes in muscle mass. Nutr Metab 13:64

REGULATION (EC) No 1924/2006 of the European Parliment and of the Council of 20 December 2006 on nutrition and health claims made on foods, lastly amended by Regulation (EU) No 1047/2012 (2006)

Salmean YA, Segal MS, Palii SP et al (2015) Fiber supplementation lowers plasma p-cresol in chronic kidney disease patients. J Ren Nutr 25:316–320

Schlemmer U, Frølich W, Prieto RM et al (2009) Phytate in foods and significance for humans: food sources, intake, processing, bioavailability, protective role and analysis. Mol Nutr Food Res 53:S330–S375

Scialla JJ, Appel LJ, Wolf M et al (2012) Plant protein intake is associated with fibroblast growth factor 23 and serum bicarbonate levels in patients with chronic kidney disease: the Chronic Renal Insufficiency Cohort study. J Ren Nutr 22:379–388

Sirich TL, Plummer NS, Gardner CD et al (2014) Effect of increasing dietary fiber on plasma levels of colon-derived solutes in hemodialysis patients. Clin J Am Soc Nephrol 9:1603–1610

St Peter WL, Wazny LD, Weinhandl ED (2018) Phosphate-binder use in US dialysis patients: prevalence, costs, evidence, and policies. Am J Kidney Dis 71:246–253

U.S. Renal Data System (2017) USRDS annual data report: Epidemiology of kidney disease in the United States. https://www.usrds.org/adr.aspx. Accessed 23 Nov 2018

Vanholder R, Schepers E, Pletinck A et al (2014) The uremic toxicity of indoxyl sulfate and p-cresyl sulfate: a systematic review. J Am Soc Nephrol 25:1897–1907

Viguiliouk E, Blanco Mejia S, Kendall CW et al (2017) Can pulses play a role in improving cardiometabolic health? Evidence from systematic reviews and meta-analyses. Ann N Y Acad Sci 1392:43–57

van Vliet S, Burd NA, van Loon LJ (2015) The skeletal muscle anabolic response to plant- versus animal-based protein consumption. J Nutr 145:1981–1991

WHO/FAO/UNU (2007) Expert consultation on protein and amino acid requirements in humans. (2007) WHO Technical Report series, No. 935

Young VR, Pellett PL (1994) Plant proteins in relation to human protein and amino acid nutrition. Am J Clin Nutr 59(5 Suppl):1203S–1212S

# Chapter 7
# Whole Pulses and Pulse Fiber: Modulating Gastrointestinal Function and the Microbiome

Wendy J. Dahl and Melissa M. Alvarez

**Abstract** Pulses are nutrient-dense foods that are high in dietary fiber. Although intakes are low for those populations consuming a Western diet, some traditional diets in parts of South America and Africa provide higher intakes of pulses. Pulses, given their high fiber content, would be expected to modulate gastrointestinal function. Research has demonstrated that the consumption of pulses and foods containing pulse fibers increases fecal weight which improves laxation. The effect of pulse and pulse fiber intake on stool frequency varies with the target population. Healthy young adults demonstrate little change, whereas patient populations, particularly those with infrequency, show increased stool frequency with pulse fiber intake. Whole pulses and pulse fibers provide non-digestible carbohydrate substrate for colonic fermentation, which contributes to gastrointestinal symptoms, especially flatulence, although reported symptoms are often mild. The provision of carbohydrate substrate (oligosaccharides, resistant start and non-starch polysaccharides) to the colonic microbiota may impact products of fermentation (e.g. acetate, propionate and butyrate) as well as the microbiota profile. Chickpea intake has been shown to have beneficial effects, specifically suppressing proteolytic bacteria while enhancing butyrate producers. Research is needed to explore the human health effects of pulse intake through the modulation of the microbiota and its metabolites.

**Keywords** Pulses · Legumes · Fiber · Microbiota · Microbiome · Stool frequency · Gastrointestinal symptoms · Stool weight · Oligosaccharide · α-galactoside

W. J. Dahl (✉) · M. M. Alvarez
Food Science and Human Nutrition Department, University of Florida, Gainesville, FL, USA
e-mail: wdahl@ufl.edu; malvarez16@ufl.edu

© Springer Nature Switzerland AG 2019
W. J. Dahl (ed.), *Health Benefits of Pulses*,
https://doi.org/10.1007/978-3-030-12763-3_7

## 7.1   Introduction

Higher fiber diets reduce the risk of a number of chronic diseases including cardiovascular disease (Threapleton et al. 2013), diabetes (Yao et al. 2014), kidney disease (Mirmiran et al. 2018) and some forms of cancer (Liu et al. 2015). However, fiber intakes are considered low in comparison to recommendations in populations consuming a Western diet, such as in the United States (Reicks et al. 2014), Canada (Kirkpatrick and Tarasuk 2008), and Europe (Murphy et al. 2012). Similarly, Asian countries such as Japan (Murakami et al. 2017) and China (Guo et al. 2017) have lower fiber intakes. In contrast, fiber intakes remain high in parts of Africa (Jariseta et al. 2012), particularly rural Africa (Alemayehu et al. 2011).

Legumes, including pulses (dried beans, dried peas and lentils), are recommended for the promotion of health due to their favorable nutrient profile (USDHHS and USDA 2015). Given the dietary fiber contents of pulses, higher intakes of pulses are correlated with higher fiber intakes in adults (Mudryj et al. 2012) and in children (Mudryj et al. 2016). Unfortunately, pulse intake in 18 countries from seven regions of the world (Africa, South and Southeast Asia, the Middle East, Europe, North America, and South America) was estimated to be only 60 g per day on average (Miller et al. 2017) which would contribute little to total fiber intake. It might be expected that in countries consuming a Mediterranean diet that traditionally includes legumes, pulse consumption would be higher. However, the SUN cohort study in Spain, a 10-year prospective study of university-educated adults, reported a baseline intake of legumes of only 21.5 ± 15.6 g/day, and showed a slight decrease over 10 years to 20.0 ± 14.7 g/day in 2009 (de la Fuente-Arrillaga et al. 2016). This intake is surprisingly similar to the Supplémentation en Vitamines et Minéraux Antioxidants cohort study conducted in France, which showed low legume intake overall, with lowest and highest tertiles consuming 20.2 g/day and 24.7 g/day, respectively (Diallo et al. 2016).

## 7.2   Defining Fiber

The many definitions of fiber have recently been reviewed (Stephen et al. 2017). However, the CODEX definition is intended to harmonize countries in this respect, and a method in line with the definition for the determination of total dietary fiber, insoluble fiber and soluble fiber has been validated in foods (McCleary et al. 2012). Within the CODEX definition, fiber is defined as "[e]dible carbohydrate polymers naturally occurring in the food as consumed" (FAO/WHO 2010), which refers to foods such as whole pulses. In contrast, most isolated pulse fibers would be considered to be "carbohydrate polymers, which have been obtained from food raw material by physical, enzymatic or chemical means and which have been shown to have a physiological effect of benefit to health as demonstrated by generally accepted scientific evidence to competent authorities" (FAO/WHO 2010). Within the Health Canada definition of fiber, "physiological effect" is defined and includes: "improves laxation or regularity by increasing stool bulk; reduces blood total and/or low-density lipoprotein cholesterol levels; reduces post-prandial blood glucose and/or insulin levels; [and] provides energy-yielding metabolites through colonic fermentation (http://www.hc-sc.gc.ca/). It is important to note that analytical methods for the determination of fiber have evolved over the years, hence cross-sectional, prospective, and interventional studies may state fiber values analyzed or calculated using differing methodologies, and thus may not be directly comparable (Dahl and Stewart 2015).

## 7.3 Fiber in Pulses

The average fiber content of a serving of pulses exceeds that which is provided by recommended serving sizes of most whole grain foods, fruits, vegetables, nuts, and seeds (USDA 2018). As reviewed by Tosh and Yada (2010), per 100 g of raw, dry weight, dry beans provide 23–32 g, chickpeas 18–22 g, lentils 18–20 g, and dry peas 14–26 g of fiber. Cooked pulses (boiled and drained) generally contain from 7 to 10 g of fiber per 100 g (USDA 2018). The fiber and macronutrient contents of commonly consumed pulses are shown in Table 7.1. In general, the contribution of insoluble fiber by far exceeds that of soluble fiber in most pulses, with 10–28 g of insoluble fiber per 100 g of raw seeds versus 2–9 g of soluble fiber (Tosh and Yada 2010).

The components of pulse fiber vary within the seed. The plant cell wall material of pulses contains primarily cellulose, hemicellulose and pectins, with the hulls of peas and beans containing higher levels of cellulose (Tosh and Yada 2010). Pulses contain oligosaccharides, specifically the α-galactosides, raffinose, stachyose and verbascose (Guillon and Champ 2002). Ciceritol, a galactosyl cyclitol, is found in

**Table 7.1** Nutrient contents of cooked pulses per 100 g fresh weight (USDA 2018)

| | Energy | Protein | Fat | Carbohydrates | Fiber |
|---|---|---|---|---|---|
| | kcal | g | g | g | g |
| Chickpeas | 164 | 8.9 | 2.6 | 27.4 | 7.6 |
| Lentils | 114 | 9.0 | 0.4 | 19.5 | 7.9 |
| Broadbeans | 110 | 7.6 | 0.4 | 19.7 | 5.4 |
| Green split peas | 116 | 8.3 | 0.4 | 20.5 | 8.3 |
| Cowpeas | 94 | 3.2 | 0.4 | 19.7 | 5.0 |
| Pigeon peas | 121 | 6.7 | 0.4 | 23.3 | 6.7 |
| Lupins | 116 | 15.6 | 2.9 | 9.3 | 2.8 |
| Kidney beans | 123 | 9.5 | 0.2 | 21.9 | 9.3 |
| Pinto beans | 162 | 9.3 | 0.5 | 30.9 | 5.4 |
| Black beans | 132 | 8.9 | 0.5 | 23.7 | 8.7 |
| White beans | 142 | 9.0 | 0.6 | 25.8 | 10.4 |

chickpeas (Quemener and Brillouet 1983) and lentils (Bernabe et al. 1993). Contents of oligosaccharides vary with pulse type but are generally estimated to be 2–10 g/100 g dry weight (Guillon and Champ 2002).

Pulses, depending on processing and cooking, provide a significant amount of resistant starch. Resistant starch is defined as starch that resists digestion in the human small intestine and passes into the colon (Higgins 2004), and from a human nutrition perspective, is often considered to be dietary fiber. The resistant starch contents of a variety of pulses have been analyzed by in vitro and in vivo methods. The resistant starch contents of cooked legumes were determined to be 1.89 ± 0.71 g/100 g for peas, 2.33 ± 1.23 g/100 g for common bean, 2.23 ± 1.15 g/100 g for chickpeas, and 2.46 ± 0.16 g/100 g for lentils, from 63% to 77% less than the raw legume (de Almeida Costa et al. 2006). In vivo analysis of the resistant starch content of cooked pulses has been shown to be significantly correlated with in vitro findings. In a study of cooked white beans, 16.5% of the ingested starch was shown to be resistant, reaching the terminal ileum, similar to the 17.1% for in vitro analysis (Noah et al. 1998). In an in vivo study of individuals with ileostomies, 22% of the starch content of red lentils escaped digestion in the small intestine (Wolever et al. 1986). Most of the starch resisting digestion is enclosed in cell walls and is RS1 (physically inaccessible starch). Beans, such as kidney, white and pinto, contain alpha-amylase inhibitors (Moreno et al. 1990) and thus have the potential to exhibit reduced starch digestion and increased starch provision to the colon. However, recommended preparation and cooking methods for beans inactivate these peptides. Raw or inadequately heat-treated beans and bean fractions provide alpha-amylase inhibitor activity and also retain their lectin activity, which can lead to deleterious gastrointestinal and systematic effects with consumption (Vasconcelos and Oliveira 2004).

## 7.4  Pulses and Gastrointestinal Function

The effects of fibers on gastrointestinal function can be assessed by measuring stool weight, stool frequency, intestinal transit time, and stool form. Stool weight is the measure commonly used to determine fecal bulking capacity, i.e. increase in fecal weight per gram of fiber intake. Stool frequency is an indicator of laxation, with low stool frequency associated with symptoms of constipation. This measure is included in the current diagnostic criteria for constipation (Rome Foundation 2006). Typical stool frequencies for those consuming a Western diet are generally between 3 stools/ week and 3 stools/day (Mitsuhashi et al. 2017). Gastrointestinal transit time can be measured directly using various methods including dyes (Compher et al. 2007), radio-opaque markers (Cummings et al. 1976), motility capsules (Saad and Hasler 2011), and more recently, magnetic resonance imaging (MRI) marker capsules (Chaddock et al. 2014), or indirectly using subjective stool form methods, such as the Bristol Stool Form Scale, a validated proxy for transit time (Riegler and Esposito 2001; Saad et al. 2010). Stool form is a much more sensitive indicator of constipation compared to stool frequency (Markland et al. 2013). Accepted physiological effects for fiber, specifically defining laxation, differ among counties. The U.S. Food and Drug Administration is currently assessing fiber efficacy studies using stool frequency as an outcome, and not the traditionally accepted outcome of stool bulking (increase in stool wet weight) as a physiological effect of fiber (FDA and USHHS 2016). In contrast, the Health Canada definition states that dietary fiber "improves laxation or regularity by increasing stool bulk" (Health Canada 2017).

Consuming foods with fiber within the plant matrix and with higher levels of insoluble fiber and lignin, positively impacts laxation. For example, cereal fiber contributes to stool bulking, decreases gastrointestinal transit time, and increases stool frequency (de Vries et al. 2015). The mean fecal bulking capacity of wheat fiber was 3.7 ± 0.09 g/day; wheat fiber increased fecal dry stool weight by 0.75 ± 0.03 g/day, somewhat less than for wheat bran (Muller-Lissner 1988). A significant effect was seen for stool frequency, an increase of 0.004 ± 0.002 stools/day per g for wheat fiber intake (de Vries et al. 2015). Given the high fiber content of whole pulses and their fiber fractions, studies have been undertaken to determine their effects on stool weight, stool frequency, and transit time.

### 7.4.1   Whole Pulses

A number of studies have examined the effect of pulses on laxation in adults, and the studies vary in the type of pulse fed (Table 7.2). Haricot beans (Leeds et al. 1982), kidney beans (Fleming et al. 1985), lentils (Stephen et al. 1995), chickpeas (Dahl et al. 2014; Murty et al. 2010), and spray-dried pulse powders (Veenstra et al. 2010) have been examined. Most of the studies involved the addition of pulses to the usual diet with one study designed as a full feeding trial (Stephen et al. 1995). Fecal bulking was examined in three trials (Fleming et al. 1985; Leeds et al. 1982; Stephen et al. 1995), stool frequency in five trials (Dahl et al. 2014; Fleming et al. 1985; Leeds et al. 1982; Murty et al. 2010; Veenstra et al. 2010), stool consistency in two trials (Murty et al. 2010; Veenstra et al. 2010), and transit time in two trials (Fleming et al. 1985; Stephen et al. 1995) (See Table 7.2).

Leeds et al. (1982) examined the effect of substituting 230 g of haricot beans (99 g dry weight) into the diets of eight women. Dietary fiber intake increased by 27–49 g/day from a baseline intake of 22 g/day. Stool frequency increased from 1.0 to 1.2 stools/day and fecal output from 115 ± 15 to 150 ± 14 g/day. These researchers also assessed transit time using continuous and single meal methodology; however, these results were inconclusive.

Fleming et al. (1985) published a report on the effect of bean intake on colonic function and fermentation. They examined fecal output, stool frequency, and intestinal transit time comparing the usual diet and with the addition of 100 g dry weight of red kidney beans per day. They compared healthy individuals, habitual bean consumers (three, 6-oz servings/week for the last 2 years) and infrequent consumers (no more than two, 6-oz servings per month). The study included a 9-day

**Table 7.2** Studies evaluating pulses and pulse fiber and gastrointestinal function

| Author (year) country | Study design | N (M/F) | Mean age (range) | Fiber (g/day) | Stool frequency | Stool weight | Gastrointestinal symptoms |
|---|---|---|---|---|---|---|---|
| Borresen et al. (2016) United States | 4-week period randomized parallel single-blind | 29 (12,7) | Control: 64 ± 14; Navy: 59 ± 12 | Control: NR; Navy bean flour: 9 + background diet | NR[a] | NR | Measured but no statistical analysis |
| Borresen et al. (2017) United States | 4-week period randomized parallel single-blind | 38 (19,19) | 10 ± 1 (8–13) | Control: 16 ± 6; NBP: 20 ± 5 | NR | NR | Measured but no statistical analysis |
| Dahl et al. (2003) Canada | 4-week periods non-randomized pre-post | 114 (34,80) | 83.9 ± 9.4 (49–103) | Control: energy matched; Pea hull: 3.1 + background diet | NS[b] | NR | NR |
| Dahl et al. (2014) Canada | 3-week periods randomized controlled, crossover | 12 (7,5) | 25.6 ± 8.7 (18–65) | Control: energy matched; Chickpea: 11.1 + background diet | NS | NR | NR |
| Fleming et al. (1985) United States | 23-day periods non-randomized pre-post | 12 (12,0) | (21–25) | Control: 33.3 ± 11.5; Kidney bean: 41.7 ± 9.3 | NS | ↑ | NR |
| Granito et al. (2005) Venezuela | 6-day periods non-randomized | 10 (0,10) | (25–40) | White bean (cooked): NR | NS | NR | ↓ flatulence with fermented beans vs cooked beans |
| Guédon et al. (1996) France | 3-week periods randomized diet-controlled | 6 (6,0) | (22–28) | Pea hull: 15 g total (g fiber NR) | NR | NR | Qualitative report of well tolerated, without clinical effects |
| Leeds et al. (1982) United Kingdom | 14-day; 10-day period pre-post | 8 (0,8) | (21–36) | Control: 22; Haricot: 49 | ↑ | ↑ | ↑ flatulence |
| Murty et al. (2010) Australia | 4, 12, 4-week periods non-randomized crossover | 42 (16,34) | (30–70) | Control: 24.3; Chickpea: 28.6; Control: 21.9 | NR | NR | ↑ flatulence |

| | | | | | | | |
|---|---|---|---|---|---|---|---|
| Salmean et al. (2015) United States | 2-week, 4-week periods pre-post | 13 (6,7) | 65 ± 3 | Control: 16.6 ± 1.7 Pea hull: 26.5 ± 2.4 | ↑ | NR | NR |
| Stephen et al. (1995) Canada | 3-week periods non-randomized diet-controlled crossover | 9 (9,0) | (18–50) | Control: NR Lentil: control +11.8 | NR | ↑ | NR |
| Veenstra et al. (2010) Canada | 4-week periods randomized double-blind placebo-controlled crossover | 79 (79,0) | 28.1 ± 5.1 | Potato: +3.5 Chickpea: +19.9 Lentil: +14.6 Green pea:+18.4 | NS | NR | ↑ flatulence severity (chickpea, lentil) ↑ bloating occurrence (lentil) ↑ cramping (chickpea, green pea) |
| Winham and Hutchins (2011) United States (3 trials) | 8-week periods randomized 2 crossover 1 parallel | Pinto/black-eyed pea: 17 Navy: 29 | 42 | Pinto: 23 ± 1.6 Black-eyed pea: 20 ± 1.6 Navy: 26 ± 1.5 Carrot control: 21 ± 1.3 Baseline: 19 ± 1.0 | NR | NR | ↑ flatulence |

[a]NR not reported
[b]NS not significant

baseline (usual diet), a 23-day intervention (cooked kidney bean given in a standardized breakfast), followed by a 23-day washout (usual diet). During the washout, the habitual intake participants consumed three cups of legumes per day, whereas the infrequent consumers had no intake of legumes. Five, 3-day fecal collections were made during intervention and washout. Intestinal transit time by dye marker was carried out three times in each study period, and three, 3-day diet records were collected. The provision of 100 g/day of kidney beans resulted in a significantly higher fecal weight (594 ± 36 g/72 h) vs. the control diet (516 ± 37 g/72 h). Overall, there was no change in defecation frequency (1.2 ± 0.1 stools/day, no beans; 1.2 ± 0.1 stools/day, beans) or intestinal transit time (41.7 ± 3.3 h, no bean; 41.1 ± 2.8 h, bean). Fiber intake was 41.7 ± 9.3 g/day during the intervention, compared to 33.3 ± 11.5 g/day during the washout.

The effects of green lentils on colonic function was examined in nine healthy men (Stephen et al. 1995). In a randomized, crossover design, participants consumed a controlled, weight maintenance, Western diet for 3 weeks and a similar diet containing 130 g/day of green lentils providing 11.8 g of dietary fiber. Mean transit time was determined using radio-opaque markers. Fecal weight was higher in the lentil period, 189 ± 17 g/day vs. 131 ± 13 g/day during the control, which represented a 5-g increase in stool weight for each gram of lentil fiber consumed. This fecal bulking capacity is similar to reports for wheat bran (Stephen et al. 1986) and higher than what was reported for wheat fiber in general (de Vries et al. 2015). However, with the consumption of lentils, mean transit time did not change in the healthy young men studied, and stool frequency was not reported.

Two trials have reported the effects of chickpea intake on laxation. In a crossover trial, the addition of 200 g of canned chickpeas to the usual diet of 12 healthy adults resulted in no change in stool frequency (Dahl et al. 2014). Murty et al. (2010) conducted a 20-week study examining the effects of chickpea intake on gastrointestinal function and symptoms as outcomes. Participants consumed a minimum of four, 300-g cans of chickpeas per week for 12 weeks in a study design with a 4-week baseline and a 4-week washout. Stool form was assessed using the Bristol Stool Form Scale. Stool frequency, ease of defecation, frequency of flatulence, and perceived bowel health were assessed. Using weighed food records with chickpea intake (105–119 g of canned chickpeas per day), fiber increased from 24.3 g/day to only 28.6 g/day. Although participants perceived improved stool frequency and softer stools, these outcomes were not significantly different, whereas flatulence increased.

One trial examined pulse flours and laxation. The effect of 100 g of spray-dried chickpea, lentil, and green field pea flours on gastrointestinal function in healthy men was investigated (Veenstra et al. 2010). With the addition of up to 19.9 g of fiber per day, no changes in stool frequency were noted. In addition, no changes in stool consistency were seen for chickpea or green pea, but a decrease in stool consistency was demonstrated with lentils. However, the interpretation of this effect is difficult, due to the lack of description of the scale used to describe stool form.

## 7.4.2   Pulse Fibers

Pulse fiber fractions have also been investigated to determine their effects on laxation (Table 7.2). Guédon et al. (1996) examined the effects of pea hull fiber and carrot fiber on colonic motility in six young men. The addition of 15 g of pea hull fiber was well tolerated with no change in daily stool frequency or stool consistency and little effect on colonic motor function. Pea fiber and fructo-oligosaccharides (FOS) were compared using a liquid diet (enteral formula) containing no fiber in ten healthy adults (Whelan et al. 2005). Stool frequency was higher on the fiber-supplemented liquid diet (0.9 ± 0.3 stools/day) compared to the fiber-free diet (0.6 ± 0.2 stools/day). Although the fiber-supplemented diet provided 27.9 g of fiber per day, there was no significant difference in fecal weights for the fiber supplemented diet (73.2 ± 37.5 g/day) and the fiber-free diet (43.8 ± 30.1 g/day). Both liquid diets exhibited lower fecal weights than baseline when subjects were consuming their usual diets (127.5 ± 71.2 g/day, baseline; 132.4 ± 68.5 g/day, washout). The report did not specify the type of pea fiber provided, but the authors' suggestion that the fiber was highly fermentable suggests it may have been a pea cotyledon fiber (Whelan et al. 2005).

In patient populations, the effect of pulse fibers on laxation has been evaluated. In a pilot study of children with constipation, consuming two snacks per day containing pea hull fiber along with inulin-supplemented beverages significantly increased stool frequency (Flogan and Dahl 2010). However, given that two fibers were provided, it is not possible to determine the contribution of the pea fiber to stool frequency. Two additional studies which examined consumption of snack foods fortified with pea hull by adults with chronic kidney disease, demonstrated increased stool frequency (Salmean et al. 2015, 2013). In the first study, pea hull fiber was used in combination with other added fibers, increasing fiber intake by 23 g/day and resulted in an increase in stool frequency from 1.2 ± 0.2 per day to 1.6 ± 0.2 per day (Salmean et al. 2013). As foods with a variety of fibers were provided, it is not possible to determine the contribution of pea hull fiber alone. However, in a second study, these same researchers compared the effects of control muffins (no added fiber) to muffins fortified with 15 g/day of pea hull, provided to participants for 4 weeks (Salmean et al. 2015). This level of pea hull fiber supplementation resulted in reported stool frequency increasing from 1.4 ± 0.2 per day to 1.9 ± 0.3 per day. Pea hull fiber (4 g/day) was added to foods of long term care residents and resulted in increased stool frequency, particularly those with low frequency of less than ten stools per month (Dahl et al. 2003).

The research suggests that pulses generally increase fecal weight but may not increase stool frequency or decrease transit time. Lack of an effect on stool frequency may be due to the population studied, as healthy adults with normal transit and typical stool frequency may not demonstrate these changes, whereas patient populations may. These findings suggest that when isolated pulse fibers are tested in healthy individuals, fecal bulking capacity may be the most appropriate, quantitative indicator of the fiber's effect on laxation.

## 7.5 Pulses and Gastrointestinal Symptoms

A long recognized side effect of pulse consumption is flatulence (Burr 1967), and this continues to be a barrier to consumption (Desrochers and Brauer 2001). Gas production, leading to flatulence, has been attributed to the oligosaccharide contents of pulses (Rackis 1975). Pulse oligosaccharides, specifically raffinose, stachyose and verbascose, are thought to undergo rapid and complete fermentation in the colon, as do other oligosaccharides (Macfarlane et al. 2008), and thus contribute to gas production and subsequent flatulence. Evidence for increased digestive symptoms has been demonstrated with feeding of up to 10 g/day of oligosaccharides from soy (Bouhnik et al. 2004). Similarly, the provision of 5 g of raffinose per day resulted in a significant increase in flatulence and bloating (Dahl et al. 2014). However in this same study, during the period where subjects consumed canned chickpeas containing very low levels of $\alpha$-galactosides, significantly higher flatulence was reported compared to during the control period. In vitro data support that soluble fiber in beans, in addition to the $\alpha$-galactosides, provides substrate for fermentation by the colonic microbiota (Granito et al. 2001). In addition, in vitro fermentation of different beans has demonstrated that the polysaccharides and resistant starch under anaerobic conditions produce short chain fatty acids (SCFA) and gases (Campos-Vega et al. 2009). As suggested by Hellendoorn (1969), and as these more recent reports provide evidence, gas and flatulence following pulse consumption results from the fermentation of all non-digestible constituents contained in pulses, including oligosaccharides, resistant starch, and non-starch polysaccharides. However, somewhat less gas and flatulence may result from pulses that are soaked (with water discarded), germinated, or fermented as these processes decrease the $\alpha$-galactosides content (Kaczmarska et al. 2017; Oboh et al. 2000).

The effect of consuming whole pulses and pulse fiber fractions on gastrointestinal symptoms has been investigated (Table 7.2). Of the nine studies examining gastrointestinal symptoms with pulse intake, three examined haricot/white navy beans (Granito et al. 2005; Leeds et al. 1982; Winham and Hutchins 2011), two studied navy bean powder (Borresen et al. 2016, 2017), one tested black-eyed and pinto beans (Winham and Hutchins 2011), one evaluated pinto beans (Winham and Hutchins 2011), one study reported on chickpea (Dahl et al. 2014), and one study tested chickpea, lentil, and green field pea (Veenstra et al. 2010) (Table 7.2).

In a study of eight women, vegetables and meat were substituted with 230 g of haricot beans for 14 days and compared to the usual diet (Leeds et al. 1982). Subjects noted an increase in flatulence, and three reported abdominal discomfort. Borresen et al. (2016) investigated the addition of navy bean powder (35 g/day) in colorectal cancer survivors and assessed tolerance using a gastrointestinal health questionnaire, and showed no major gastrointestinal symptoms. These same researchers, in a non-randomized study examining the effect of cooked navy bean powder (17.5 g/day) on cholesterol lowering in children, also assessed changes in symptoms such as flatulence (Borresen et al. 2017). Reported gastrointestinal symptoms were minimal, similar to the children in the control group. However, in these three investigations, no statistical analyses were presented.

In a study of ten women, 6-day intakes of 45 g/day of cooked white navy beans vs. cooked and fermented white navy beans (separated by a 2-week washout) were compared to evaluate the effects on gastrointestinal symptoms and function (Granito et al. 2005). Previous research reported a significant decrease in dietary fiber content of beans by in vitro fermentation (Granito et al. 2001), thus lower symptoms were expected. Analysis of the bean products showed that cooking and fermentation eliminated the oligosaccharides, and decreased the resistant starch and insoluble fiber contents. The only significant difference was less flatulence with the fermented beans. No differences were seen in bloating, noises, abdominal pain, nausea, or diarrhea.

Three studies evaluated the effect of one-half cup/day of pulses on perception of flatulence (Winham and Hutchins 2011). In the first study, participants (n = 17) were randomized to consume one-half cup/day of black-eyed peas, pinto beans, or carrot each for 8-week period. In study 2, 29 participants consumed baked beans or carrots each for 8 weeks. In the third study, a parallel design, 40 participants consumed one-half cup of pinto beans or control soup. The same gastrointestinal symptom questionnaire was used for all three studies. Pulses contributed to increased flatulence, with the exception of black-eyed peas, whereas only pinto beans contributed to bloating.

In a randomized, double-blind, controlled trial of 21 healthy men, gastrointestinal symptoms, including flatulence and abdominal discomfort, were examined (Veenstra et al. 2010). During 28-day intervention periods, spray-dried powders of chickpea, lentil, and green field pea (100 g/day) provided 19.9 g (4.4 g RS; 1.9 g $\alpha$-galactosides), 14.6 g (4.8 g RS; 2.6 g $\alpha$-galactosides), and 18.4 g (5.2 g RS; 3.5 g $\alpha$-galactosides) of dietary fiber, respectively. A visual analogue scale was used to assess symptoms. Statistically significant increases in flatulence with chickpea and lentil were demonstrated. No changes in cramping, bloating, urgency, or problems with defecation were noted with the single exception of a transient increase in bloating for green field pea.

In a crossover trial, Dahl et al. (2014) reported increased flatulence and bloating with 200 g of canned chickpea incorporated into the participants' usual diet. In another study examining chickpea (140 g cooked per day) on metabolic parameters, of the 21 participants assigned to the chickpea diet, one withdrew due to abdominal discomfort (Nestel et al. 2004); however, gastrointestinal symptoms were not systematically assessed.

These studies confirm that flatulence is a common side effect of pulse consumption. It has been stated that gastrointestinal effects, specifically flatulence, decrease over time (Winham and Hutchins 2011). As suggested by Leeds et al. (1982), adaption of the microbiota to the provision of a fermentable substrate does occur; however, the adaptation likely involves increased fermentation. With increased fermentation, one would not expect a decrease in gas production unless a specific change occurred whereby substrate utilization was switched to non-gas-producing bacteria groups. Only one study examined short or long term adaptation of pulses. With kidney bean intake, no decrease in gas excretion over time was found, although subjective tolerance may have improved (O'Donnell and Fleming

1984). Winham and Hutchins (2011) reported a perceived decrease in symptoms over time. However, this observation may have been an artifact of the questionnaire used to assess a change in gastrointestinal symptoms over the previous week.

Pulses are included in the foods to avoid in the FODMAPS (low fermentable oligo-, di-, and monosaccharides and polyols) diet, which has been evaluated for its efficacy in decreasing gastrointestinal symptoms in irritable bowel syndrome (IBS) patients. Numerous systematic reviews have been carried out to assess the efficacy of the FODMAPS diet for symptom management (Altobelli et al. 2017; Krogsgaard et al. 2017; Rao et al. 2015; Schumann et al. 2018). These analyses conclude that higher quality randomized controlled trials are needed to assess the efficacy of the FODMAP diet, as well as its long-term safety. The FODMAP diet requires the restriction of a number of health-promoting foods such as pulses. High doses of monosaccharides, disaccharides, and polyols may contribute to an increase in small intestinal water and gas production (Staudacher and Whelan 2017); however, symptoms induced by the levels of these sugars and sugar alcohols in foods such as pulses have not been examined. Given the low level of oligosaccharides that a serving of pulses would provide, the appropriateness of exclusion in this diet is questionable. In addition, canned pulses may have very low contents of oligosaccharides (Fernando et al. 2010), as do soaked and well-cooked, fermented, and sprouted pulses (Kaczmarska et al. 2017; Oboh et al. 2000).

## 7.6   Pulses and Pulse Fibers and Microbiota

Pulse fiber, whether it be intact in whole pulses or isolated by dehulling, is considered dietary fiber and provides substrate to the colonic microbiota. Often dietary recommendations refer to pulses being a source of soluble fiber in reference to health benefits, but as with cereal fiber, the association with prevention of chronic disease suggests insoluble fiber may have a more significant role (Cho et al. 2013; Ye et al. 2012). However, given the high total fiber contents of pulses, the soluble fiber levels of pulses are physiologically significant and contribute to their association with health (Ha et al. 2014). Total fiber, including the insoluble and soluble fractions, may be related to reduced disease risk through the modulation of microbiota, its activities and, potentially, inflammation (Dahl et al. 2017).

Little work has been carried out related to the colonic fermentation of pulse fibers and their effects on the colonic microbiota profile. Stephen et al. (1995) fed green lentils, providing about 12 g of dietary fiber. About 75% of the lentil fiber was fermented when consumed by healthy adults, including 52% of the cellulose, 97% of the arabinose, and 61% of the xylose. Dominianni et al. (2015) examined the association of dietary fiber intake and microbiome, and specifically examined bean fiber which showed a greater abundance of Actinobacteria phylum, specifically Bifidobacteriales. Fernando et al. (2010) carried out a 9-week, cross-over trial examining the effect of 200 g of canned chickpeas and 5 g raffinose, the main oligosaccharide component of chickpeas, on fecal microbiota. With raffinose, a small increase in *Bifidobacterium* compared to the control was noted. With both chickpea and raffinose intake, a significant increase in *Faecalibacterium prausnitzii* (*F. prausnitzii*) was reported. This is of interest given that this bacterium is a butyrate producer, and counts of this bacteria seem to be lower in patients with one of a number of disease states (Jiang et al. 2017; Liu et al. 2017; Takahashi et al. 2016). *F. prausnitzii* is also enhanced with weight loss (Remely et al. 2015). Thus, *F. prausnitzii* may be associated with a more balanced, healthful microbiota. During chickpea intake, the number of study participants showing *Clostridium histolyticum – Clostridium lituseburense,* which include proteolytic bacteria, also decreased. Detection of high ammonia-producers dropped from 83% on the control foods to 42% of individuals when consuming chickpea. No change in bacterial species diversity was seen with either the chickpea or raffinose interventions in these healthy participants.

In a 4-week, randomized, single-blind, parallel design study of colon cancer survivors (n = 29), cooked navy bean powder (35 g/day), heat-stabilized rice bran (30 g/day), and a macronutrient control were evaluated for their effects on microbiota and fermentation metabolites (Sheflin et al. 2017). Fecal samples were taken at baseline, 14 and 28 days. Feeding either substrate resulted in increased bacterial diversity. However, the navy bean powder did not alter the ratio of Firmicutes to Bacteriodetes, whereas rice bran did. Stool community structure was assessed with principal component analysis. No changes were noted with either treatment. Navy bean powder suppressed *Bacteriodes fragilis* (days 14 and 28), an unclassified Lachnobacterium, and an unclassified Lachnospira and Coprococcus increased compared to baseline.

An older, but interesting study used fluorescent in situ hybridization (FISH) methodology to compare microbiota changes with an enteral formula containing pea fiber and FOS and an enteral formula devoid of fiber (Whelan et al. 2005). The researchers completed a re-analysis to specifically investigate butyrate producers, i.e. *Roseburia* and *Fecalibacterium* spp. (Benus et al. 2010). Decreases were seen in all bacterial species with both the fiber-free and fiber formulas compared to usual diet, with the exception of *Bifidobacterium* spp., which increased with fiber-supplementation. This is not surprising given that FOS has a demonstrated bifidogenic effect (Vandeputte et al. 2017). Large decreases in both *F. prausnitzii* and *Roseburia intestinalis* were seen with both the fiber-free and fiber-supplemented formulas, and *Bacteriodes* decreased with the fibre-free diet (Benus et al. 2010).

It has been suggested that the products of fermentation may be as important, or more important, than minor changes in the microbiota profile (Dahl et al. 2017). SCFA provide energy. Specifically, butyrate is utilized by the colonocytes, acetate is oxidized systematically, and propionate is metabolized in the liver (Macfarlane and Macfarlane 2012). In addition, SCFA may have a significant role in disease modulation (Gill et al. 2018). Studies to date showed no changes in fecal SCFA for chickpea (Fernando et al. 2010), navy bean powder (Sheflin et al. 2017), or kidney beans (Fleming et al. 1985). It is important to note, however, as greater than 95% of SCFA produced in the colon are absorbed (Macfarlane and Macfarlane 2012), fecal losses may not necessarily reflect production and absorption.

## 7.7 Summary

Human studies of pulses and pulse fibers have demonstrated stool bulking but inconsistent effects on stool frequency, a common finding when testing fibers on individuals with normal stool frequency. Very few studies have examined the effect of whole pulses and pulse fibers on transit time or its proxy, stool form, although this outcome is associated with microbiota profile and its metabolism. As microbiome is increasingly associated with health outcomes, further research on the impacts of pulses and pulse fiber is needed.

# References

Alemayehu AA, Abebe Y, Gibson RS (2011) A 24-h recall does not provide a valid estimate of absolute nutrient intakes for rural women in southern Ethiopia. Nutrition 27:919–924

Altobelli E, Del Negro V, Angeletti P et al. (2017) Low-FODMAP diet improves irritable bowel syndrome symptoms: a meta-analysis. Nutrients 9. doi:https://doi.org/10.3390/nu9090940

Benus RF, van der Werf TS, Welling GW et al (2010) Association between Faecalibacterium prausnitzii and dietary fibre in colonic fermentation in healthy human subjects. Br J Nutr 104:693–700

Bernabe M, Fenwick R, Frias J et al (1993) Determination, by NMR spectroscopy, of the structure of ciceritol, a pseudotrisaccharide isolated from lentils. J Agric Food Chem 41:870–872

Borresen EC, Brown DG, Harbison G et al (2016) A randomized controlled trial to increase navy bean or rice bran consumption in colorectal cancer survivors. Nutr Cancer 68:1269–1280

Borresen EC, Jenkins-Puccetti N, Schmitz K et al (2017) A pilot randomized controlled clinical trial to assess tolerance and efficacy of navy bean and rice bran supplementation for lowering cholesterol in children. Glob Pediatr Health 4:2333794x17694231. https://doi.org/10.1177/23 33794x17694231

Bouhnik Y, Raskine L, Simoneau G et al (2004) The capacity of nondigestible carbohydrates to stimulate fecal bifidobacteria in healthy humans: a double-blind, randomized, placebo-controlled, parallel-group, dose-response relation study. Am J Clin Nutr 80:1658–1664

Burr HK (1967) Making legumes more acceptable. Paper presented at the Western Expt. Sta. Coll. Conf., Albany

Campos-Vega R, Reynoso-Camacho R, Pedraza-Aboytes G et al (2009) Chemical composition and in vitro polysaccharide fermentation of different beans (*Phaseolus vulgaris* L.). J Food Sci 74:T59–T65

Chaddock G, Lam C, Hoad CL et al (2014) Novel MRI tests of orocecal transit time and whole gut transit time: studies in normal subjects. Neurogastroenterol Motil 26:205–214

Cho SS, Qi L, Fahey GC Jr et al (2013) Consumption of cereal fiber, mixtures of whole grains and bran, and whole grains and risk reduction in type 2 diabetes, obesity, and cardiovascular disease. Am J Clin Nutr 98:594–619

Compher C, Rubesin S, Kinosian B et al (2007) Noninvasive measurement of transit time in short bowel syndrome. J Parenter Enter Nutr 31:240–245

Cummings JH, Jenkins DJ, Wiggins HS (1976) Measurement of the mean transit time of dietary residue through the human gut. Gut 17:210–218

Dahl WJ, Stewart ML (2015) Position of the Academy of Nutrition and Dietetics: health implications of dietary fiber. J Acad Nutr Diet 115:1861–1870

Dahl WJ, Whiting SJ, Healey A et al (2003) Increased stool frequency occurs when finely processed pea hull fiber is added to usual foods consumed by elderly residents in long-term care. J Am Diet Assoc 103:1199–1202

Dahl WJ, Hanifi A, Zello GA et al (2014) Gastrointestinal tolerance to daily canned chickpea intake. Can J Diet Pract Res 75:218–221

Dahl WJ, Agro NC, Eliasson ÅM et al (2017) Health benefits of fiber fermentation. J Am Coll Nutr 36:127–136

de Almeida Costa GE, da Silva Q-MK, Pissini Machado Reis SM et al (2006) Chemical composition, dietary fibre and resistant starch contents of raw and cooked pea, common bean, chickpea and lentil legumes. Food Chem 94:327–330

de la Fuente-Arrillaga C, Zazpe I, Santiago S et al (2016) Beneficial changes in food consumption and nutrient intake after 10 years of follow-up in a Mediterranean cohort: the SUN project. BMC Public Health 16:203. https://doi.org/10.1186/s12889-016-2739-0

de Vries J, Miller PE, Verbeke K (2015) Effects of cereal fiber on bowel function: a systematic review of intervention trials. World J Gastroenterol 21:8952–8963

Desrochers N, Brauer PM (2001) Legume promotion in counselling: an e-mail survey of dietitians. Can J Diet Pract Res 62:193–198

Diallo A, Deschasaux M, Galan P et al (2016) Associations between fruit, vegetable and legume intakes and prostate cancer risk: results from the prospective Supplementation en Vitamines et Mineraux Antioxydants (SU.VI.MAX) cohort. Br J Nutr 115:1579–1585

Dominianni C, Sinha R, Goedert JJ et al (2015) Sex, body mass index, and dietary fiber intake influence the human gut microbiome. PLoS One 10(4):e0124599. https://doi.org/10.1371/journal.pone.0124599

Fernando WM, Hill JE, Zello GA et al (2010) Diets supplemented with chickpea or its main oligosaccharide component raffinose modify faecal microbial composition in healthy adults. Benefic Microbes 1:197–207

Fleming SE, O'Donnell AU, Perman JA (1985) Influence of frequent and long-term bean consumption on colonic function and fermentation. Am J Clin Nutr 41:909–918

Flogan C, Dahl WJ (2010) Fiber fortification improves gastrointestinal function and decreases energy intake in children with a history of constipation. Infant Child Adolesc Nutr 2:312–317

Food and Drug Administration; US Department of Health and Human Services (2016) Scientific review of the beneficial physiological effects of non-digestible carbohydrate for meeting the FDA definition of dietary fiber. https://www.fda.gov/downloads/Food/LabelingNutrition/UCM610139.pdf. Accessed 21 Nov 2018

Gill PA, van Zelm MC, Muir JG et al (2018) Review article: short chain fatty acids as potential therapeutic agents in human gastrointestinal and inflammatory disorders. Aliment Pharmacol Ther 48:15–34

Granito M, Champ M, David A et al (2001) Identification of gas-producing components in different varieties of *Phaseolus vulgaris* by in vitro fermentation. J Sci Food Agric 81:543–550

Granito M, Michel C, Frías J et al (2005) Fermented *Phaseolus vulgaris*: acceptability and intestinal effects. Eur Food Res Technol 220:182–186

Guedon CP, Ducrotte JM, Antoine P et al (1996) Does chronic supplementation of the diet with dietary fibre extracted from pea or carrot affect colonic motility in man? Br J Nutr 76(1):51–61

Guillon F, Champ M-J (2002) Carbohydrate fractions of legumes: uses in human nutrition and potential for health. Br J Nutr 88(S3):293–306

Guo QY, Zhao LY, He YN et al (2017) Survey on dietary nutrients intake of Chinese residents between 2010 and 2012. Zhonghua Yu Fang Yi Xue Za Zhi 51:519–522

Ha V, Sievenpiper JL, de Souza RJ et al (2014) Effect of dietary pulse intake on established therapeutic lipid targets for cardiovascular risk reduction: a systematic review and meta-analysis of randomized controlled trials. CMAJ 186:E252–E262

Health Canada (2017) Policy for labelling and advertising of dietary fibre-containing food products. https://www.canada.ca/en/health-canada/services/publications/food-nutrition/labelling-advertising-dietary-fibre-food-products.html. Accessed 23 Nov 2018

Hellendoorn E (1969) Intestinal effects following ingestion of beans. Food Technol 23:795–799

Higgins JA (2004) Resistant starch: metabolic effects and potential health benefits. J AOAC Int 87:761–768

Jariseta ZR, Dary O, Fiedler JL et al (2012) Comparison of estimates of the nutrient density of the diet of women and children in Uganda by Household Consumption and Expenditures Surveys (HCES) and 24-hour recall. Food Nutr Bull 33(3 Suppl):S199–S207

Jiang S, Xie S, Lv D et al (2017) Alteration of the gut microbiota in Chinese population with chronic kidney disease. Sci Rep 7:2870. https://doi.org/10.1038/s41598-017-02989-2

Joint FAO/WHO Food Standards Programme, Secretariat of the CODEX Alimentarius Commission (2010) CODEX Alimentarius (CODEX) guidelines on nutrition labeling CAC/GL 2–1985 as last amended 2010. FAO, Rome

Kaczmarska KT, Chandra-Hioe MV, Zabaras D et al (2017) Effect of germination and fermentation on carbohydrate composition of Australian sweet lupin and soybean seeds and flours. J Agric Food Chem 65:10064–10073

Kirkpatrick SI, Tarasuk V (2008) Food insecurity is associated with nutrient inadequacies among Canadian adults and adolescents. J Nutr 138:604–612

Krogsgaard LR, Lyngesen M, Bytzer P (2017) Systematic review: quality of trials on the symptomatic effects of the low FODMAP diet for irritable bowel syndrome. Aliment Pharmacol Ther 45:1506–1513

Leeds A, Khumalo T, Ndaba N et al (1982) Haricot beans, transit time and stool weight. J Plant Foods 4:33–41

Liu L, Wang S, Liu J (2015) Fiber consumption and all-cause, cardiovascular, and cancer mortalities: a systematic review and meta-analysis of cohort studies. Mol Nutr Food Res 59:139–146

Liu HN, Wu H, Chen YZ et al (2017) Altered molecular signature of intestinal microbiota in irritable bowel syndrome patients compared with healthy controls: a systematic review and meta-analysis. Dig Liver Dis 49:331–337

Macfarlane GT, Macfarlane S (2012) Bacteria, colonic fermentation, and gastrointestinal health. J AOAC Int 95:50–60

Macfarlane GT, Steed H, Macfarlane S (2008) Bacterial metabolism and health-related effects of galacto-oligosaccharides and other prebiotics. J Appl Microbiol 104:305–344

Markland AD, Palsson O, Goode PS et al (2013) Association of low dietary intake of fiber and liquids with constipation: evidence from the National Health and Nutrition Examination Survey. Am J Gastroenterol 108:796–803

McCleary BV, DeVries JW, Rader JI et al (2012) Determination of insoluble, soluble, and total dietary fiber (CODEX definition) by enzymatic-gravimetric method and liquid chromatography: collaborative study. J AOAC Int 95:824–844

Miller V, Mente A, Dehghan M et al (2017) Fruit, vegetable, and legume intake, and cardiovascular disease and deaths in 18 countries (PURE): a prospective cohort study. Lancet 390:2037–2049

Mirmiran P, Yuzbashian E, Asghari G et al (2018) Dietary fibre intake in relation to the risk of incident chronic kidney disease. Br J Nutr 119:479–485

Mitsuhashi S, Ballou S, Jiang ZG et al (2017) Characterizing normal bowel frequency and consistency in a representative sample of adults in the United States (NHANES). Am J Gastroenterol 113:115. https://doi.org/10.1038/ajg.2017.213

Moreno J, Altabella T, Chrispeels MJ (1990) Characterization of alpha-amylase-inhibitor, a lectin-like protein in the seeds of Phaseolus vulgaris. Plant Physiol 92:703–709

Mudryj AN, Yu N, Hartman TJ et al (2012) Pulse consumption in Canadian adults influences nutrient intakes. Br J Nutr 108(Suppl 1):S27–S36

Mudryj AN, Aukema HM, Fieldhouse P et al (2016) Nutrient and food group intakes of Manitoba children and youth: a population-based analysis by pulse and soy consumption status. Can J Diet Pract Res 77:189–194

Muller-Lissner SA (1988) Effect of wheat bran on weight of stool and gastrointestinal transit time: a meta analysis. Br Med J (Clin Res Ed) 296:615–617

Murakami K, Livingstone MB, Okubo H et al (2017) Energy density of the diets of Japanese adults in relation to food and nutrient intake and general and abdominal obesity: a cross-sectional analysis from the 2012 National Health and Nutrition Survey, Japan. Br J Nutr 117:161–169

Murphy N, Norat T, Ferrari P et al (2012) Dietary fibre intake and risks of cancers of the colon and rectum in the European prospective investigation into cancer and nutrition (EPIC). PLoS One 7:e39361. https://doi.org/10.1371/journal.pone.0039361

Murty CM, Pittaway JK, Ball MJ (2010) Chickpea supplementation in an Australian diet affects food choice, satiety and bowel health. Appetite 54:282–288

Nestel P, Cehun M, Chronopoulos A (2004) Effects of long-term consumption and single meals of chickpeas on plasma glucose, insulin, and triacylglycerol concentrations. Am J Clin Nutr 79:390–395

Noah L, Guillon F, Bouchet B et al (1998) Digestion of carbohydrate from white beans (*Phaseolus vulgaris* L.) in healthy humans. J Nutr 128:977–985

O'Donnell A, Fleming S (1984) Influence of frequent and long-term consumption of legume seeds on excretion of intestinal gases. Am J Clin Nutr 40:48–57

Oboh HA, Muzquiz M, Burbano C et al (2000) Effect of soaking, cooking and germination on the oligosaccharide content of selected Nigerian legume seeds. Plant Foods Hum Nutr 55:97–110

Quemener B, Brillouet J-M (1983) Ciceritol, a pinitol digalactoside form seeds of chickpea, lentil and white lupin. Phytochemistry 22:1745–1751

Rackis JJ (1975) Oligosaccharides of food legumes: alpha-galactosidase activity and the flatus problem. ACS Publications. Northern Regional Research Laboratory, U.S. Department of Agriculture, Peoria

Rao SS, Yu S, Fedewa A (2015) Systematic review: dietary fibre and FODMAP-restricted diet in the management of constipation and irritable bowel syndrome. Aliment Pharmacol Ther 41:1256–1270

Reicks M, Jonnalagadda S, Albertson AM et al (2014) Total dietary fiber intakes in the US population are related to whole grain consumption: results from the National Health and Nutrition Examination Survey 2009 to 2010. Nutr Res 34:226–234

Remely M, Tesar I, Hippe B et al (2015) Gut microbiota composition correlates with changes in body fat content due to weight loss. Benefic Microbes 6:431–439

Riegler G, Esposito I (2001) Bristol scale stool form. A still valid help in medical practice and clinical research. Tech Coloproctol 5:163–164

Rome Foundation (2006) Guidelines – Rome III diagnostic criteria for functional gastrointestinal disorders. J Gastrointest Liver Dis 15:307–312

Saad RJ, Hasler WL (2011) A technical review and clinical assessment of the wireless motility capsule. Gastroenterol Hepatol 7:795–804

Saad RJ, Rao SS, Koch KL et al (2010) Do stool form and frequency correlate with whole-gut and colonic transit? Results from a multicenter study in constipated individuals and healthy controls. Am J Gastroenterol 105:403–411

Salmean YA, Zello GA, Dahl WJ (2013) Foods with added fiber improve stool frequency in individuals with chronic kidney disease with no impact on appetite or overall quality of life. BMC Res Notes 6:510. https://doi.org/10.1186/1756-0500-6-510

Salmean YA, Segal MS, Palii SP et al (2015) Fiber supplementation lowers plasma p-cresol in chronic kidney disease patients. J Ren Nutr 25:316–320

Schumann D, Klose P, Lauche R et al (2018) Low fermentable, oligo-, di-, mono-saccharides and polyol diet in the treatment of irritable bowel syndrome: a systematic review and meta-analysis. Nutrition 45:24–31

Sheflin AM, Borresen EC, Kirkwood JS et al (2017) Dietary supplementation with rice bran or navy bean alters gut bacterial metabolism in colorectal cancer survivors. Mol Nutr Food Res 61. doi:https://doi.org/10.1002/mnfr.201500905

Staudacher HM, Whelan K (2017) The low FODMAP diet: recent advances in understanding its mechanisms and efficacy in IBS. Gut 66:1517–1527

Stephen AM, Wiggins HS, Englyst HN et al (1986) The effect of age, sex and level of intake of dietary fibre from wheat on large-bowel function in thirty healthy subjects. Br J Nutr 56:349–361

Stephen AM, Dahl WJ, Sieber GM et al (1995) Effect of green lentils on colonic function, nitrogen balance, and serum lipids in healthy human subjects. Am J Clin Nutr 62:1261–1267

Stephen AM, Champ MM, Cloran SJ et al (2017) Dietary fibre in Europe: current state of knowledge on definitions, sources, recommendations, intakes and relationships to health. Nutr Res Rev 30:149–190

Takahashi K, Nishida A, Fujimoto T et al (2016) Reduced abundance of butyrate-producing bacteria species in the fecal microbial community in Crohn's disease. Digestion 93:59–65

Threapleton DE, Greenwood DC, Evans CE et al (2013) Dietary fibre intake and risk of cardiovascular disease: systematic review and meta-analysis. BMJ 347:f6879. https://doi.org/10.1136/bmj.f6879

Tosh SM, Yada S (2010) Dietary fibres in pulse seeds and fractions: characterization, functional attributes, and applications. Food Res Int 43:450–460

U.S. Department of Agriculture (2018) Agricultural Research Service, Nutrient Data Laboratory. USDA National Nutrient Database for Standard Reference, Legacy. Version Current: April 2018. Internet: /nea/bhnrc/ndl

U.S. Department of Health and Human Services, US Department of Agriculture (2015) 2015–2020 dietary guidelines for Americans. 8th edition. http://health.gov/dietaryguidelines/2015/guidelines/. Accessed 23 Nov 2018

Vandeputte D, Falony G, Vieira-Silva S et al (2017) Prebiotic inulin-type fructans induce specific changes in the human gut microbiota. Gut 66:1968–1974

Vasconcelos IM, Oliveira JT (2004) Antinutritional properties of plant lectins. Toxicon 44:385–403

Veenstra J, Duncan A, Cryne C et al (2010) Effect of pulse consumption on perceived flatulence and gastrointestinal function in healthy males. Food Res Int 43:553–559

Whelan K, Judd PA, Preedy VR et al (2005) Fructooligosaccharides and fiber partially prevent the alterations in fecal microbiota and short-chain fatty acid concentrations caused by standard enteral formula in healthy humans. J Nutr 135:1896–1902

Winham DM, Hutchins AM (2011) Perceptions of flatulence from bean consumption among adults in 3 feeding studies. Nutr J 10:128. https://doi.org/10.1186/1475-2891-10-128

Wolever TM, Cohen Z, Thompson LU et al (1986) Ileal loss of available carbohydrate in man: comparison of a breath hydrogen method with direct measurement using a human ileostomy model. Am J Gastroenterol 81:115–122

Yao B, Fang H, Xu W et al (2014) Dietary fiber intake and risk of type 2 diabetes: a dose-response analysis of prospective studies. Eur J Epidemiol 29:79–88

Ye EQ, Chacko SA, Chou EL et al (2012) Greater whole-grain intake is associated with lower risk of type 2 diabetes, cardiovascular disease, and weight gain. J Nutr 142:1304–1313

# Chapter 8
# Potential Health Promoting Properties of Isoflavones, Saponins, Proanthocyanidins, and Other Phytonutrients in Pulses

**Yavuz Yagiz and Liwei Gu**

**Abstract** This chapter reviews the structure, concentration, absorption, and health promoting activities of phytonutrients in pulses. The phenolic phytonutrients in pulses include isoflavones, flavan-3-ols, proanthocyanidins, hydroxycinnamic acids, and flavanols. A major non-phenol phytonutrient is saponins. The bioactivities of pulse phytonutrients which may have a beneficial role in cardiovascular disease, obesity, diabetes, cancer, inflammation, and neurodegenerative disease are summarized. Gaps of knowledge in the previous research are suggested and future research directions are proposed.

**Keywords** Pulses · Legumes · Phytonutrients · Isoflavones · Saponins · Flavonols · Proanthocyanidins · Hydrocinnamic acids · Bioavailability · Anti-inflammatory

## 8.1 Introduction

Pulses contain several classes of phytonutrients with diverse structures that may have health benefits. Phytonutrients are secondary metabolites in pulses. The total content of phytonutrients in pulses is typically less than 3–5% w/w. These compounds may have health-promoting properties related to cardiovascular diseases, cancers, inflammation, diabetes, and neurodegenerative diseases. Many phytonutrients in pulses are polyphenols with potent antioxidant capacity to scavenge harmful free radicals and toxic carbonyls. Some of these phytonutrients may impact human health by altering the diversity and composition of microbiota in human gut.

Phytonutrients in pulses can be divided into phenolics and non-phenol compounds. Major phenolic phytonutrients include isoflavones, flavan-3-ols,

---

Y. Yagiz · L. Gu (✉)
Food Science and Human Nutrition Department, University of Florida, Gainesville, FL, USA
e-mail: yavuzy@ufl.edu; lgu@ufl.edu

© Springer Nature Switzerland AG 2019
W. J. Dahl (ed.), *Health Benefits of Pulses*,
https://doi.org/10.1007/978-3-030-12763-3_8

**Table 8.1** Contents of total phenolics, total flavonoids, and total proanthocyanidins in pulses (Xu and Chang 2007)

|  | Total phenolic compound (mg gallic acid equivalents/g) | Total flavonoid (mg catechin equivalents/g) | Proanthocyanidins (mg catechin equivalents/g) |
|---|---|---|---|
| Pea | 1.53 | 0.39 | 1.71 |
| Chickpea | 1.81 | 3.16 | 1.85 |
| Lentil | 6.56 | 2.21 | 8.78 |
| Black bean | 6.89 | 3.21 | 6.74 |

proanthocyanidins, hydroxycinnamic acids, and flavanols (Table 8.1). Major non-phenol phytonutrients are saponins.

## 8.2  Isoflavones

Isoflavones are unique phytonutrients in pulses, better known as phytoestrogens. This is because absorbed isoflavones bind with estrogen receptor $\alpha$ and $\beta$ to function as estrogen agonists or antagonists. The relative affinities of isoflavones on human estrogen receptor $\beta$ is about 0.04% for daidzein and 7.4% for genistein in comparison with 17$\beta$-estradiol in vitro (Muthyala et al. 2004). Pulses are the only dietary sources of isoflavones besides soybean.

### 8.2.1  Structures and Concentration

The structures of isoflavones in pulses are shown in Fig. 8.1. Majority of the isoflavones in pulses exist in their glycoside form, including daidzin (daidzein 7-*O*-β-D-glucoside) and genistin (genistein 7-*O*-β-D-glucoside). Some of these glycosides are hydrolyzed during cooking or fermentation to lose their glucose moiety. Isoflavone glycosides are often hydrolyzed using acids or enzymes and the resultant isoflavone aglycones are quantified on high performance liquid chromatography (HPLC). The concentration of isoflavones in different pulses are listed in Table 8.2. Common beans have the highest concentration of isoflavones, followed by chickpea and pea, with lentils having lower concentrations. Formonogetin is a major isoflavones in lentils and chickpea but not in pea or bean. Biochanin-A appears to be unique in chickpea.

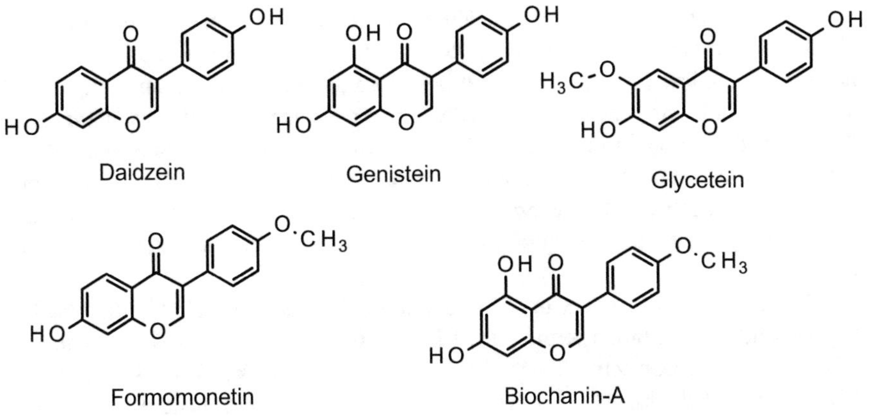

**Fig. 8.1** Structures of isoflavones in pulses

**Table 8.2** Contents of isoflavones in pulses (Bhagwat et al. 2008; Delgado-Zamarreño et al. 2012)

|  | Pea | Lentil | Bean | Chickpea |
|---|---|---|---|---|
|  | µg/g |  |  |  |
| Daidzein[a] | 3.3 | 0.1 | 2.9 | 2.3 |
| Genistein[a] | 1.1 | 0.5 | 3.0 | 0.6 |
| Glycetein[a] | n.d. | n.d. | n.d. | 2.2 |
| Daidzin | n.a. | 10.0 | n.a. | n.a. |
| Genistin | n.a. | 3.8 | n.a. | n.a. |
| Formononetin | n.a. | 6.3 | n.a. | 4.0 |
| Biochanin-A | n.a. | n.a. | n.a. | 3.2 |
| Total isoflavone[a] | 4.4 | 0.6 | 5.9 | 3.8 |

n.d. not detected, n.a. no data available
[a]Includes both aglycone and glycosides

## 8.2.2  Absorption and Metabolism

Isoflavone glycosides are not absorbed directly. They are hydrolyzed by β-glycosidase present in the brush border of the mammalian small intestine and some of the isoflavone glycosides are hydrolyzed by microbiota in the large intestine. The resultant isoflavone aglycones are absorbed into intestinal epithelial cells through passive diffusion due to the lack of transporters. Phase I metabolism of isoflavones in the intestine and liver is minimal. Isoflavones undergo phase II metabolism to conjugate with sulphates or/and glucuronides. Some of isoflavone sulfates or glucuronides are effluxed by multidrug resistance proteins in enterocytes back to the gut lumen. Absorbed isoflavones and their phase-II conjugates enter liver through portal vein. Additional phase II metabolism take place in the liver. A portion of isoflavones conjugates in liver are effluxed by multidrug resistance proteins into bile duct, from there they re-enter the small intestine through enterohepatic circulation.

Unabsorbed isoflavones are degraded by microbiota in colon into various metabolites. S-equol is a microbial metabolite of daidzein. It has drawn significant attention during the last 10 years because it is a more potent than daidzein. S-equol had a binding affinity of 3.2% of estradiol on human estrogen receptor β compared with 0.04% for daidzein (Muthyala et al. 2004). About 59% of vegetarians and 25% of non-vegetarian adults have the capacity to metabolize daidzein into S-equol. They are the so-called "equol producers". It has been suggested that isoflavones have different biological effects on equol producers and non-producers (Setchell and Cole 2006).

Absorption rates of isoflavones are much higher than other phytonutrients. The $C_{max}$ of daidzein in human serum reached 1.3–2.6 μM at $T_{max}$ of 6.0–8.5 h. The $C_{max}$ of genistein in human serum reached 1.6–4.1 μM at $T_{max}$ of 5.5–7.8 h (Cassidy et al. 2006). About 62% ingested daidzein and 22% of ingested genistein are excreted into urine (King and Bursill 1998). The absorption behavior of formononetin and biochanin A appear similar to daidzein and genistein (Tsunoda et al. 2002).

### 8.2.3 Potential Health Promoting Properties

#### 8.2.3.1 Cancer

Isoflavones are associated with reducing the risk of breast and prostate cancers owing to their estrogenic activities. The lower incidence of breast cancers in Asian women comparing with Western women has been attributed to higher intake of soy isoflavones. Decreased risk of breast cancer in Asian women but not Western women is associated with isoflavones intake (Chen et al. 2014). Women in the highest quintile of isoflavones intake had a 22% reduced risk of breast cancer compared to those with a median intake of 1.15 mg/day (Jaceldo-Siegl et al. 2015). A meta-analysis of observational studies concluded that genistein and daidzein intake was associated with a decreased risk of prostate cancers (He et al. 2015).

Possible mechanisms of isoflavones have been investigated in animal and cell cancer models. Oral daidzein or equol at a human equivalent dose suppressed the growth of both DMBA-induced mammary tumors and human MCF-7 breast cancer xenografts in mice (Liu et al. 2012). Dietary exposure to genistein induced PTEN expression in mammary epithelial cells in vivo and in vitro, which may suggest a breast cancer preventive mechanism (Rahal and Simmen 2010). Genistein was also shown to inhibit DNA methylation and increases expression of tumor suppressor genes in human breast cancer cells (Xie et al. 2014). Formononetin directly inhibited proliferation and blocked the oncogenic signaling pathways in breast cancer cells (Wu et al. 2015a, b). Genistein has been shown to inhibit human prostate cancer cell detachment, invasion, growth, and metastasis (Pavese et al. 2014). Formononetin promotes cell cycle arrest via downregulation of Akt/Cyclin D1/CDK4 in human prostate cancer cells (Li et al. 2014). S-equol inhibited prostate cancer growth in vitro and in vivo, though activating the AKT/FOXO3a pathway (Lu et al. 2016).

### 8.2.3.2 Cardiometabolic Risk

A pooled analysis of three US cohort studies concluded that the intake of isoflavones was associated with a modestly lower T2D risk in US men and women who typically consumed low-to-moderate amounts of soy foods (Ding et al. 2016). Isoflavones at a dose of 435 mg/day for 2 months significantly reduced total cholesterol, triglyceride, and LDL-cholesterol while increasing HDL-cholesterol in patients with type 2 diabetes (Chi et al. 2016).

Animal models elucidate some possible mechanisms of isoflavones related to cardiometabolic risk factors. Formononetin suppressed the adipogenic differentiation of 3T3-L1 fibroblasts through down-regulation of key adipogenic markers. Formononetin supplemented diet for 12 weeks inhibited the development of obesity in mice by attenuating high fat diet-induced body weight gain and visceral fat accumulation. Formononetin increased energy expenditure and protected against high fat diet-induced dyslipidaemia (Gautam et al. 2017). Genistein for 24 weeks (0.5 g/kg diet) alleviated hepatic steatosis by lowering serum and hepatic cholesterol and lipid peroxidation levels, and hepatic heme oxygenase 1 protein levels in ApoE(−/−) mice (Jeon et al. 2014). A recent study showed that S-equol, a microbial metabolites of daidzein, protected against streptozotocin-induced hyperglycemia by increasing $\beta$-cell function in male mice (Horiuchi et al. 2017).

### 8.2.3.3 Menopausal Symptoms

A meta-analysis summarized that isoflavones reduced the frequency of hot flushes and co-occurring symptoms during the menopausal transition and postmenopause, without serious side-effects (Chen et al. 2015). A randomized, double-blind, placebo-controlled study showed that a low-dose (25 mg/day) of isoflavones was effective to alleviate menopausal symptoms of depression and insomnia in middle-aged women (Hirose et al. 2016). Genistein supplementation at 30 mg/day reduced the number of hot flushes by 51% in postmenopausal women. Women receiving the genistein also reported significantly fewer hot flushes per day and a decrease in total duration of hot flushes per day at week 12 vs. placebo (Evans et al. 2011).

### 8.2.3.4 Neurodegenerative Disease

There is little data to support an association of isoflavone intake and neurodegenerative diseases. In an Alzheimer's disease mouse model, genistein resulted in a remarkable and rapid improvement cognitive functions including hippocampal learning, recognition memory, implicit memory, and odor discrimination. Genistein decreased associated Amyloid-$\beta$ levels in brain, reduced the number and the area of amyloid plaques (confirmed in vivo by positron emission tomography) as well as microglial reactivity (Bonet-Costa et al. 2016). Amyloid-$\beta$ contributes the development of Alzheimer's disease by oxidative damage of the neurons. Formononetin and genistein effectively inhibited Amyloid-β induced neurotoxicity (Chen et al. 2017; Luo et al. 2012; Wu et al. 2015a, b). In an animal model of Parkinson's disease, genistein treatment improved learning and memory abilities in Morris water maze (Arbabi et al. 2016). Biochanin A or daidzein inhibited microglial activation and subsequent release of toxic pro-inflammatory factors in microglial cell, suggesting it may play a role in the prevention of Parkinson's disease (Chinta et al. 2013).

## 8.3 Saponins

Saponins are secondary metabolites, amphiphilic, heat-stable, glycosidic compounds which are naturally present in a wide variety of edible pulses including lentils, chickpeas, and common beans.

### 8.3.1 Structures and Concentration

The general structure of saponins in pulses is shown in Fig. 8.2. Saponins are plant glycosides in which the non-sugar moiety is a steroid or a triterpenoid compound. The sugar moieties are usually mono- or oligosaccharides attached to an aglycone. The amphiphilic nature of saponins is due to the lipid soluble aglycone linked to sugar residues. The structures of saponins in pulses are variable and depend on the types and amount of sugar, the degree and position of glycosylation and structures of the ring. The major saponins present in pulses are derivatives of soyasaponins. The concentration of saponins in various pulses is listed in Table 8.3. Saponin contents in pulses range between 1 and 43 g/kg. Saponin content in chickpea (21 g/kg) is higher than other pulses such as pea (11 g/kg) and lentils (5–6.2 g/kg). Processing such as cooking and soaking have a significant impact on the concentration of saponins in pulses. For example, soaking and cooking of chickpeas and lentils reduced the saponin content of chickpea by 2–5% and of lentils by 6–12% (Ruiz et al. 1996).

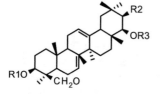

| | |
|---|---|
| Soyasapoenol A: | R1=H; R2=OH; R3=H |
| Soyasapoenol B: | R1=H; R2=H; R3=H |
| Phaseoside I: | R1=GlcA[2]-Gal[2]-Glc; R2=H; R3=Ara[2]-Glc |
| Soyasaponin I: | R1=GlcA[2]-Gal[2]-Rha; R2=H; R3=H |
| Soyasaponin II: | R1=GlcA[2]-Ara[2]-Rha; R2=H; R3=H |
| Soyasaponin III: | R1=GlcA [2]-Gal; R2=H; R3=H |
| Soyasaponin A1: | R1=GlcA[2]-Gal[2]-Glc; R2=OH; R3=Ara[3]-Glc |
| Soyasaponin A2: | R1=GlcA[2]-Gal; R2=OH; R3=Ara[3]-Glc |

**Fig. 8.2** Structures of saponins in pulses

**Table 8.3** Contents of saponins in pulses

|  | Saponin concentration g/kg dry weight |
|---|---|
| Pea[a] | 11 |
| Chickpea[a] | 21 |
| Lentil[b] | 5.0–6.2 |
| Broad bean[a] | 1 |
| Mung bean[a] | 5 |
| Butter bean[a] | 10 |
| Kidney bean[a] | 35 |
| Haricot bean[a] | 41 |
| Pigeon bean[a] | 10 |
| Balor bean[a] | 10 |
| Black eyed bean[a] | 10 |
| Navy bean[c] | 39.8 |
| Dark red kidney bean[c] | 40.6 |
| Pinto bean[c] | 41.4 |
| Black turtle soup bean[c] | 42.8 |

[a]Data source Ridout et al. (1988)
[b]Data source Fenwick and Oakenfull (1983)
[c]Data source Drumm et al. (1990)

## 8.3.2   Absorption and Metabolism

Saponins are poorly absorbed in the human small intestine. A portion of saponins form insoluble large mixed micelles with bile acids and cholesterol. Some of saponins are hydrolyzed by intestinal bacteria to aglycones. In vivo experiments on mice, rats, and chicks showed that ingested saponins were not detected in the blood as saponins or aglycones. The ingested saponins were not found in the stomach or small intestine. However, they were detected in the large intestine in the forms of aglycones and sugars. This suggests that saponins were metabolized by the gut microflora of chicks, rats, and mice to release sugars and aglycone (Gestetner et al. 1968). Incubation of human fecal bacteria anaerobically with soyasaponin (10 mmol) at 37 °C for 48 h resulted in a disappearance of soyasaponin I with first order reaction kinetics. Research showed that human gut microbial enzymes degraded soyasaponin I to soyasaponenol B and smaller soyasaponins with fewer sugars attached to the aglycone (Hu et al. 2004).

## 8.3.3   Potential Health Promoting Properties

### 8.3.3.1   Cancer

Saponins have antioxidant properties and possess direct and selective cytotoxicity against cancer cells as do many compounds. The total consumption of pulses is approximately 8–18 g/day in Japan as opposed to 3–10 g/day in some western countries (Rao and Sung 1995). Several epidemical studies suggested that the lower colon cancer rates in East Asian populations in comparison with Western populations may be in part due to the consumption of foods with higher content of saponins (Dunn 1975; Messina et al. 1994; Miller et al. 1994; Tominaga 1999).

Animal and cell studies have explored potential mechanisms of saponins in cancer models. A rat study providing a diet containing a very high level of saponin (3%) inhibited the development of azoxymethane induced preneoplastic lesions in the colon by about 67% (Koratkar and Rao 1997). Saponins extracted from soybeans inhibited the growth of colon carcinoma cells and induced cancer cell apoptosis. Bile acids promote epithelial cell proliferation; however, the saponins that bind to bile acid inhibited the cell proliferation (Rao and Sung 1995). Saponins interact with free or membrane bound sterols and secondary metabolites of bile acids (Kendall et al. 1992). Soyasaponins and aglycone were tested for growth suppression of HT-29 colon cancer cells over a concentration range of 0–50 ppm. Aglycones soyasapogenol A and B were the most effective compounds whereas the glycosidic soyasaponins were inactive. The anticancer activity of soyasaponins increased with higher lipophilicity (Gurfinkel and Rao 2003).

### 8.3.3.2   Serum Cholesterol

Saponins decrease cholesterol level by forming an insoluble complex with cholesterol and thereby, hinder its absorption in the intestine. Saponins bind to cholesterol and inhibit further cholesterol oxidation in the colon (Sidhu and Oakenfull 1986). Meta-analysis level data supports that pulse intake decreases serum low-density lipoprotein (LDL) cholesterol (Ha et al. 2014). In a human intervention study, the consumption of a diet consisting of beans, lentils, and field peas over a 7-week period significantly reduced serum LDL cholesterol and increased the excretion of fecal bile acids which may be in part due to saponins (Duane 1997).

Animal experiments have shown similar cholesterol lowering effects. In rats, saponin decreased liver and aorta cholesterol concentrations from 7.27 to 6.26 mmol/g and from 3.9 and 3.6 to 3.3 mmol/g, respectively (Sautier et al. 1979). Whole navy beans containing saponins decreased blood cholesterol in rats whereas navy beans without saponins did not show any cholesterol-lowering effect. This result suggested that the saponins in navy bean are responsible to significantly lower plasma cholesterol concentration (Kozuharov et al. 1986). Similarly, isolated chickpea saponins decreased plasma cholesterol concentrations in rats and humans (Oakenfull and Sidhu 1984). In rats, soyasaponins I and βg extracted from lentil reduced the plasma cholesterol, LDL-cholesterol, while increasing HDL-cholesterol, bile acids level in the feces, the concentration of short chain fatty acids, and growth of *Bifidobacterium* spp. (3 log) (Micioni di Bonaventura et al. 2017). Group B soyasaponins (2.2 mmol/kg, 4w) significantly reduced plasma total cholesterol (20%), non-HDL cholesterol (33%), and triglycerides (18%) and resulted in increasing fecal excretion of bile acids and neutral sterols in hamsters (Lee et al. 2005).

## 8.4   Flavan-3-Ols and Proanthocyanidins

### 8.4.1   Structures and Concentration

Proanthocyanidins, oligomers and polymers of flavan-3-ols, are also known as condensed tannins. Structures of flavan-3-ols and proanthocyanidins in pulses are shown in Fig. 8.3. The most common flavan-3-ols in pulses are (+)-catechin and (−)-epicatechin. Proanthocyanidins consisting exclusively of (+)-catechin and (−)-epicatechin are procyanidins. Size of proanthocyanidins is described using degree of polymerization. Proanthocyanidins consisting of 2, 3, or 4 flavan-3-ols are called dimer, trimers, or tetramer. Procyanidin dimers have a total of eight isomers labelled as B1 to B8. Procyanidin trimers have three isomers, labelled as C1 to C3. All pulses contain (+)-catechin or (−)-epicatechin, however, only lentil and bean contained proanthocyanidins (Table 8.4).

### 8.4.2   Absorption and Metabolism

Catechin, epicatechin, proanthocyanidin dimers and trimers are absorbable in small intestine albeit the absorption rate is low. Absorption decreases with increased molecular weight. Absorbed flavan-3-ols undergo phase II metabolism in intestine and liver to form glucuronidated, sulfated, and methylated metabolites. Proanthocyanidins larger than tetramers are considered non-absorbable. Majority of

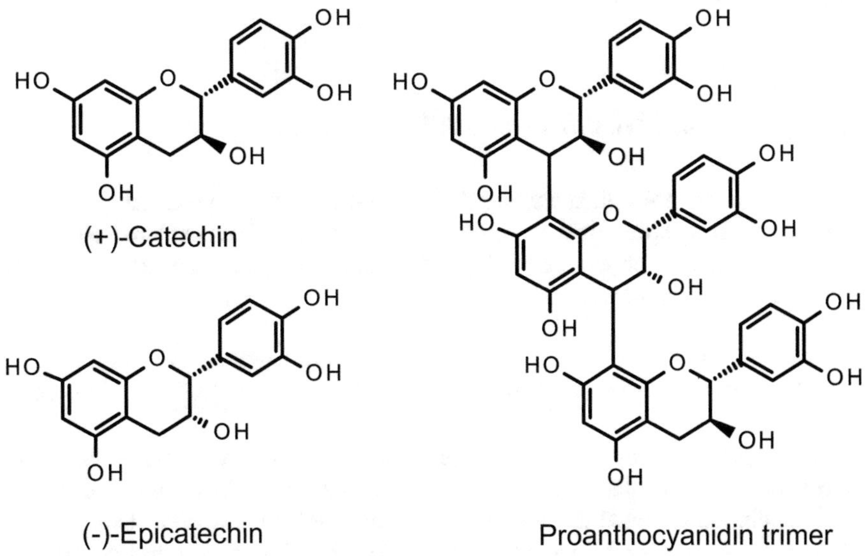

**Fig. 8.3** Structures of flavan-3-ols and condensed tannins in pulses

**Table 8.4** Contents of flavan-3-ols and proanthocyanidins in pulses (Multari et al. 2016; Nayak et al. 2011; Bittner et al. 2013)

|                                      | Pea    | Lentil | Pinto Bean | Chickpea |
| ------------------------------------ | ------ | ------ | ---------- | -------- |
|                                      | mg/kg  |        |            |          |
| (+)-catechin                         | 205    | 30.7   | 201        | 151      |
| (−)-epicatechin                      | n.d.   | n.d.   | 5.4        | 23.9     |
| Procyanidin dimers (sum of B1–B8)    | n.d.   | 230    | 274        | n.d.     |
| Procyanidin trimers (sum of C1-C3)   | n.d.   | 213    | 65.5       | n.d.     |

*n.d.* not detected

ingested flavan-3-ols and proanthocyanidins pass through the small intestine to enter the colon where they are catabolized by gut microbiota into numerous metabolites including hydroxyphenyl-γ-valerolactones, hydroxyphenyl valeric acids, hydroxyphenylpropionic acids, hydroxyphenylacetic acids, and hippuric acid (Monagas et al. 2010). These bacteria-derived phenolic acids are the predominant metabolites of flavan-3-ols and proanthocyanidins (Gu et al. 2007).

After the ingestion of a single dose of epicatechin or procyanidin B1 (1 mg EC per kg body weight), concentrations in human plasma reach peaks of 150 ng/mL and 1.9 ng/mL in about 2 h, respectively. 5-(3′,4′-dihydroxyphenyl)-valerolactone is a microbial metabolite. Its plasma peak concentration reached 300 ng/ml for epicatechin at 8 h and 200 ng/mL for procyanidin B1 at 10 h. A total of 4% ingested epicatechin were recovered in 24 h-urine whereas procyanidin B1 was not detected in urine (Wiese et al. 2015). The peak plasma concentration of procyanidin B4 was 2.13 ng/mL and mean total urinary excretion related to the administered dose was 0.008 ± 0.003% in pigs after a single dose of 10 mg/kg body weight (Bittner et al. 2014).

## 8.4.3 Potential Health Promoting Properties

Although tannins are well known for their antinutrient effects, potential health promoting effects of flavan-3-ols and proanthocyanidins have been explored. Research has been limited to animal and cell studies, and thus, cannot be extrapolated to health benefits in humans.

### 8.4.3.1 Anti-inflammatory Activity

Proanthocyanidins suppress inflammatory responses in human dendritic cells and selectively down-regulate Th1 response in naive T cells (Williams et al. 2017). Procyanidin B2 inhibited the activation of NLRP3 inflammasome and subsequent caspase-1 activation and interleukin (IL)-1β secretion in response to lipopolysaccharides (LPS) in human endothelial cells. It also attenuated LPS-induced production of reactive oxygen species (ROS) and the transcriptional activity of activator protein-1 (Yang et al. 2014). Both procyanidin B2 and C1 suppress inflammation by inhibiting LPS-induced NF-κB signaling in macrophages (Byun et al. 2013). Proanthocyanidins at a dose of 200 mg/kg per day in a rat model facilitated the recovery of pathologic damage of colon caused by recurrent colitis. It showed significant protective effect by inhibiting inflammatory cell infiltration, promoting damaged tissue repair, and reducing oxidative stress in colon (Wang et al. 2010).

### 8.4.3.2   Cancer

DNA methyltransferases is a key epigenetic enzyme for cancer growth. Procyanidin B2 in attenuated DNMT activity at IC50 of 6.88 μM and subsequently enhanced the expression of DNMT target genes, suggesting it has therapeutic value (Shilpi et al. 2015). Proanthocyanidin oligomers inhibited the proliferation but induced the apoptosis of human prostate cancer cells (Neuwirt et al. 2008). Proanthocyanidins in the diet for 9 month significantly reduced dimethylnitrosamine-induced liver tumorigenesis, carcinogenesis and mortality in male B6C3F1 mice (Ray et al. 2005). Feeding female rats diets containing 0.1–1.0% proanthocyanidins caused 72–88% inhibition of AOM-induced aberrant crypt foci (an early sign of colon cancer) formation in rats (Singletary and Meline 2001). Procyanidins are known to suppress the growth of human colorectal cancer cells by affect PI3K/Akt pathway (Choy et al. 2016).

### 8.4.3.3   Obesity and Diabetes

High fat diet for 15 weeks led to obesity and insulin resistance in C57BL/6J mice. Supplementing diet with epicatechin ameliorated the adverse effects of high fat diet, and particularly, improved insulin sensitivity (Cremonini et al. 2016). Epicatechin is thought to modulate high calorie diet induced obesity through enhancing the oxidation of fatty acids and energy expenditure in white adipose tissues (Rabadan-Chavez et al. 2016). Procyanidin B2 inhibits adipogenesis and differentiation of 3T3-L1 pre-adipocytes by targeting specific nuclear receptors in cell (Zhang et al. 2017). Dietary intake of epicatechin promoted survival in diabetic mice (50% mortality in diabetic control group vs. 8.4% in epicatechin group after 15 week of treatment) and improved skeletal muscle stress output, reduced systematic inflammation markers and serum LDL cholesterol (Si et al. 2011). The administration of proanthocyanidins at 10 mg/kg body weight in diabetic mice reduced serum level of glucose and glycosylated protein, decreased the levels of triglyceride, total cholesterol, and oxidative stress. Procyanidin oligomers showed much higher activity than polymers (Lee et al. 2008).

## 8.5  Flavonols and Hydrocinnamic Acids

### 8.5.1  Structures and Concentration

The structures of flavonols and hydrocinnamic acids in pulses are shown in Fig. 8.4. The amount of kaempferol is highest in beans followed by chickpea. The concentration of myricetin is high in chickpea and lentil. Pea and bean are the only pulses containing quercetin. Taxifolin, tyrosol and chlorogenic acid were found in pea with a concentration of 0.48, 2.11 and 260 mg/kg, respectively (Table 8.5). Processing, such as cooking and soaking, significantly impact the concentration of flavonols. For instance, thermal processing reduced the amount of kaempferol-3-glucoside and kaempferol-3-acetylglucoside in pinto beans as compared to the raw pinto beans (Xu and Chang 2009).

### 8.5.2  Absorption and Metabolism

Flavonols and hydrocinnamic acids are poorly absorbed similar to other phytonutrients. The hydrocinnamic acids in beans were absorbed 1–3 h after the consumption of beans with the maximum plasma concentrations usually less than 0.5 μmol/L. Their clearance from the blood was fast and half-life for clearance in urine was less than 2 h. The absorption rate of quercetin and kaempferol in beans were about 1–2%. The clearance of quercetin and kaempferol from blood is slow compared to the

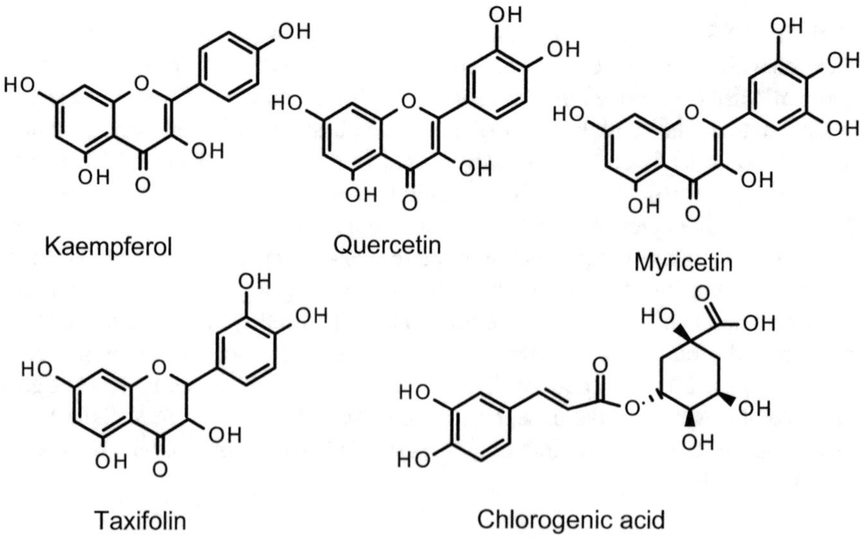

**Fig. 8.4**  Structures of flavonols and hydrocinnamic acid in pulses

**Table 8.5** Contents of flavonols and hydrocinnamic acids in pulses (Multari et al. 2016; Nayak et al. 2011; Bhagwat et al. 2014)

| | Pea | Lentil | Bean | Chickpea |
|---|---|---|---|---|
| | mg/kg | | | |
| Kaempferol | 2.74 | 2.78 | 23.5 | 18.1 |
| Myricetin | n.d. | 33.3 | 3.3 | 32.0 |
| Quercetin | 1.08 | n.a. | 2.3 | n.a. |
| Taxifolin | 0.48 | n.a. | n.a. | n.a. |
| Tyrosol | 2.11 | n.a. | n.a. | n.a. |
| Chlorogenic acid | 260[a] | n.a. | n.a. | n.a. |

*n.d.* not detected, *n.a.* no data available
[a]dry pea flour

other phenolic compounds due to longer clearance half-life of 15–20 h, therefore, these flavonols stay in blood for longer period of times. Poor absorption of flavonols and hydrocinnamic acids is partially due to efficient glucuronadation in intestine which causes the export of the glucuronidated phenolic compounds back into gut lumen. Additional glucuronidation and sulfation takes place in the liver. Following glucurodnidation and sulfation, much of the absorbed polyphenolic compounds were excreted into the bile and never reach the blood (Manach et al. 2005).

Pea has a high content of chlorogenic acid which is the ester of caffeic acid with quinic acid. After dietary intake of chlorogenic acid (250 µmol/day, 8 day) in rats, the recovery of chlorogenic acid was low (0.8%, mol/mol) in urine, and the total urinary recovery of caffeic acid and its tissular methylated metabolites did not exceed 0.5% of the dose of chlorogenic acid ingested. The microbial metabolites (57.5% mol/mol) of the chlorogenic acid intake were seen in both urine and plasma. The high abundance of microbial metabolites demonstrated that the bioavailability of the chlorogenic acid rely on its metabolism by the gut microflora (Gonthier et al. 2003).

### 8.5.3   Potential Health Promoting Properties

#### 8.5.3.1   Obesity and Diabetes

Inhibition of enzymes ($\alpha$-glucosidase and lipase) involved in carbohydrates and lipids digestion has been proposed as a strategy against diabetes and obesity. The phenolic extracts from 20 lentil varieties inhibited $\alpha$-glucosidase in the rat intestine with IC50 ranging from 23.08 to 42.15 mg/mL (Zhang et al. 2015). Similar inhibitory activities on $\alpha$-glucosidase were reported for beans (Sreerama et al. 2012). The phenolic compounds, specifically flavonols e.g. kaempferol and quercetin glycosides are the key contributors to the inhibitory activity on $\alpha$-glucosidase (Li et al. 2009). The hydrophilic extracts from 20 lentils inhibited the pancreatic lipase with $IC_{50}$ from 6.26 to 9.26 mg/mL. The most significant correlation was seen between the $IC_{50}$ values and total flavonol index (TFI) ($R^2 = -0.8802$), suggesting major contributors of lipase inhibitory activity were flavonols (Zhang et al. 2015). Similarly, quercetin or kaempferol exerted strong inhibitory activity on pancreatic lipase (Sergent et al. 2012).

Dietary intake of caffeic acid and chlorogenic acid in high-fat diet induced-obese mice were significantly reduced body weight, visceral fat mass and plasma leptin and insulin levels. They also significantly reduced triglyceride (in plasma, liver and heart) and cholesterol (in plasma, adipose tissue and heart) concentrations (Rodriguez de Sotillo and Hadley 2002). In a single human study, chlorogenic acid intake reduced early fasting glucose and insulin response in 15 overweight men during oral glucose tolerance test (OGTT) (van Dijk et al. 2009).

### 8.5.3.2 Cancer

A meta-analysis of 12 epidemiological studies concluded that a high intake of flavonols was significantly correlated to a reduced risk of gastric cancer, especially in women and smokers (Xie et al. 2016). Another meta-analysis suggested that dietary isoflavones and flavonols have a protective effect against ovarian cancer (Hua et al. 2016).

The antimutagenic and anticarcinogenic activities of flavonols are partially due to their antioxidant capacities in decreasing oxidative stress (Willett et al. 2002). Quercetin in pulses had the highest antioxidant activities 367 $\mu M$ Trolox equivalent in TEAC assay (Zhang et al. 2015). Quercetin in diet for 1 week significantly reduced the number of palpable mammary tumors in female rats (Verma et al. 1988). A single exposure to quercetin or kaempferol (1, 5, 10 $\mu M$, 4 day/14 day) or combined quercetin and kaempferol (1, 5, 10 $\mu M$, 4 day/14 day) reduced cell proliferation in two human gut cell lines HuTu-80 and Caco-2 and the PMC42 human breast cell line (Ackland et al. 2005).

## 8.6 Conclusions and Future Research Directions

Phytonutrients in pulses are considered non-essential; however, they have health promoting properties that may have a role in preventing cardiovascular disease, obesity, diabetes, cancers, inflammation, and neurodegenerative diseases. Major phenolic phytonutrients in pulses include: isoflavones, flavan-3-ols, proanthocyanidins, hydroxycinnamic acids, and flavonols. Major non-phenol phytonutrients are mainly saponins. The research on the phytonutrients in pulses are still in an early stage compared to other plant-sourced foods. Concentration and profile data of phytonutrients in pulses are incomplete and lacking. A better understanding of how cooking and processing impact the content and bioavailability of phytonutrients in pulses is needed. Human studies, exploring metabolomics and the microbiome are needed to gain a better understanding of the bioactivities of pulse phytonutrients and their effects on human health.

# References

Ackland ML, Van de Waarsenburg S, Jones R (2005) Synergistic antiproliferative action of the flavonols quercetin and kaempferol in cultured human cancer cell lines. In Vivo 19:69–76

Arbabi E, Hamidi G, Talaei SA et al (2016) Estrogen agonist genistein differentially influences the cognitive and motor disorders in an ovariectomized animal model of Parkinsonism. Iran J Basic Med Sci 19:1285–1290

Bhagwat S, Haytowitz D B, Holden JM (2008) USDA database for the isoflavone content of selected foods. https://www.ars.usda.gov/ARSUserFiles/80400525/Data/isoflav/Isoflav_R2.pdf. Accessed 21 Nov 2018

Bhagwat S, Haytowitz DB, Holden JM (2014) USDA database for the flavonoid content of selected foods. https://www.ars.usda.gov/ARSUserFiles/80400525/Data/Flav/Flav_R03-1.pdf. Accesssed 21 Nov 2018

Bittner K, Rzeppa S, Humpf HU (2013) Distribution and quantification of flavan-3-ols and procyanidins with low degree of polymerization in nuts, cereals, and legumes. J Agric Food Chem 61:9148–9154

Bittner K, Kemme T, Peters K et al (2014) Systemic absorption and metabolism of dietary procyanidin B4 in pigs. Mol Nutr Food Res 58:2261–2273

Bonet-Costa V, Herranz-Perez V, Blanco-Gandia M et al (2016) Clearing amyloid-beta through PPARgamma/ApoE activation by genistein is a treatment of experimental Alzheimer's disease. J Alzheimers Dis 51:701–711

Byun EB, Sung NY, Byun E et al (2013) The procyanidin trimer C1 inhibits LPS-induced MAPK and NF-kappaB signaling through TLR4 in macrophages. Int Immunopharmacol 15:450–456

Cassidy A, Brown JE, Hawdon A et al (2006) Factors affecting the bioavailability of soy isoflavones in humans after ingestion of physiologically relevant levels from different soy foods. J Nutr 136:45–51

Chen M, Rao Y, Zheng Y et al (2014) Association between soy isoflavone intake and breast cancer risk for pre- and post-menopausal women: a meta-analysis of epidemiological studies. PLoS One 9:e89288

Chen MN, Lin CC, Liu CF (2015) Efficacy of phytoestrogens for menopausal symptoms: a meta-analysis and systematic review. Climacteric 18:260–269

Chen L, Ou S, Zhou L et al (2017) Formononetin attenuates Abeta25-35-induced cytotoxicity in HT22 cells via PI3K/Akt signaling and non-amyloidogenic cleavage of APP. Neurosci Lett 639:36–42

Chi XX, Zhang T, Zhang DJ et al (2016) Effects of isoflavones on lipid and apolipoprotein levels in patients with type 2 diabetes in Heilongjiang Province in China. J Clin Biochem Nutr 59:134–138

Chinta SJ, Ganesan A, Reis-Rodrigues P et al (2013) Anti-inflammatory role of the isoflavone diadzein in lipopolysaccharide-stimulated microglia: implications for Parkinson's disease. Neurotox Res 23:145–153

Choy YY, Fraga M, Mackenzie GG et al (2016) The PI3K/Akt pathway is involved in procyanidin-mediated suppression of human colorectal cancer cell growth. Mol Carcinog 55:2196–2209

Cremonini E, Bettaieb A, Haj FG et al (2016) (-)-Epicatechin improves insulin sensitivity in high fat diet-fed mice. Arch Biochem Biophys 599:13–21

Delgado-Zamarreño MM, Pérez-Martín L, Bustamante-Rangel M et al (2012) Pressurized liquid extraction as a sample preparation method for the analysis of isoflavones in pulses. Anal Bioanal Chem 404:361–366

Ding M, Pan A, Manson JE et al (2016) Consumption of soy foods and isoflavones and risk of type 2 diabetes: a pooled analysis of three US cohorts. Eur J Clin Nutr 70:1381–1387

Drumm TD, Gray JI, Hosfield GL (1990) Variability in the saccharide, protein, phenolic acid and saponin contents of four market classes of edible dry beans. J Sci Food Agric 51:285–297

Duane W (1997) Effects of legume consumption on serum cholesterol, biliary lipids, and sterol metabolism in humans. J Lipid Res 38:1120–1128

Dunn JE (1975) Cancer epidemiology in populations of the United States—with emphasis on Hawaii and California—and Japan. Cancer Res 35:3240–3245

Evans M, Elliott JG, Sharma P et al (2011) The effect of synthetic genistein on menopause symptom management in healthy postmenopausal women: a multi-center, randomized, placebo-controlled study. Maturitas 68:189–196

Fenwick DE, Oakenfull D (1983) Saponin content of food plants and some prepared foods. J Sci Food Agric 34:186–191

Gautam J, Khedgikar V, Kushwaha P et al (2017) Formononetin, an isoflavone, activates AMP-activated protein kinase/beta-catenin signalling to inhibit adipogenesis and rescues C57BL/6 mice from high-fat diet-induced obesity and bone loss. Br J Nutr 117:645–661

Gestetner B, Birk Y, Tencer Y (1968) Soybean saponins: fate of ingested soybean saponins and the physiological aspect of their hemolytic activity. J Agric Food Chem 16:1031–1035

Gonthier MP, Verny MA, Besson C et al (2003) Chlorogenic acid bioavailability largely depends on its metabolism by the gut microflora in rats. J Nutr 133:1853–1859

Gu L, House SE, Rooney L et al (2007) Sorghum bran in the diet dose dependently increased the excretion of catechins and microbial-derived phenolic acids in female rats. J Agric Food Chem 55:5326–5334

Gurfinkel D, Rao A (2003) Soyasaponins: the relationship between chemical structure and colon anticarcinogenic activity. Nutr Cancer 47:24–33

Ha V, Sievenpiper JL, de Souza RJ et al (2014) Effect of dietary pulse intake on established therapeutic lipid targets for cardiovascular risk reduction: a systematic review and meta-analysis of randomized controlled trials. CMAJ 186:E252–E262

He J, Wang S, Zhou M et al (2015) Phytoestrogens and risk of prostate cancer: a meta-analysis of observational studies. World J Surg Oncol 13:231

Hirose A, Terauchi M, Akiyoshi M et al (2016) Low-dose isoflavone aglycone alleviates psychological symptoms of menopause in Japanese women: a randomized, double-blind, placebo-controlled study. Arch Gynecol Obstet 293:609–615

Horiuchi H, Usami A, Shirai R et al (2017) S-Equol activates cAMP signaling at the plasma membrane of INS-1 pancreatic beta-cells and protects against Streptozotocin-induced hyperglycemia by increasing beta-cell function in male mice. J Nutr 147:1631–1639

Hu J, Zheng YL, Hyde W et al (2004) Human fecal metabolism of soyasaponin I. J Agric Food Chem 52:2689–2696

Hua X, Yu L, You R et al (2016) Association among dietary flavonoids, flavonoid subclasses and ovarian cancer risk: a meta-analysis. PLoS One 11:e0151134

Jaceldo-Siegl K, Gatto N, Beeson L et al (2015) Intake of soy isoflavones reduces breast cancer incidence among women in North America. FASEB J 29(1 Supplement). Retrieved from http://www.fasebj.org/content/29/1_Supplement/406.5.abstract

Jeon S, Park YJ, Kwon YH (2014) Genistein alleviates the development of nonalcoholic steatohepatitis in ApoE(−/−) mice fed a high-fat diet. Mol Nutr Food Res 58:830–841

Kendall CW, Koo M, Sokoloff E et al (1992) Effect of dietary oxidized cholesterol on azoxymethane-induced colonic preneoplasia in mice. Cancer Lett 66:241–248

King RA, Bursill DB (1998) Plasma and urinary kinetics of the isoflavones daidzein and genistein after a single soy meal in humans. Am J Clin Nutr 67:867–872

Koratkar R, Rao AV (1997) Effect of soya bean saponins on azoxymethane-induced preneoplastic lesions in the colon of mice. Nutr Cancer 27:206–209

Kozuharov S, Oakenfull D, Sidhu G (1986) Navy beans and navy bean saponins lower plasma cholesterol concentrations in rats. Paper presented at the Proc. Nutr. Soc. Aust

Lee SO, Simons AL, Murphy PA et al (2005) Soyasaponins lowered plasma cholesterol and increased fecal bile acids in female golden Syrian hamsters. Exp Biol Med 230:472–478

Lee YA, Cho EJ, Yokozawa T (2008) Effects of proanthocyanidin preparations on hyperlipidemia and other biomarkers in mouse model of type 2 diabetes. J Agric Food Chem 56:7781–7789

Li H, Song F, Xing J, Tsao R et al (2009) Screening and structural characterization of $\alpha$-glucosidase inhibitors from hawthorn leaf flavonoids extract by ultrafiltration LC-DAD-MSn and SORI-CID FTICR MS. J Am Soc Mass Spectrom 20:1496–1503

Li T, Zhao X, Mo Z et al (2014) Formononetin promotes cell cycle arrest via downregulation of Akt/Cyclin D1/CDK4 in human prostate cancer cells. Cell Physiol Biochem 34:1351–1358

Liu X, Suzuki N, Santosh Laxmi YR et al (2012) Anti-breast cancer potential of daidzein in rodents. Life Sci 91:415–419

Lu Z, Zhou R, Kong Y et al (2016) S-equol, a secondary metabolite of natural anticancer isoflavone daidzein, inhibits prostate cancer growth in vitro and in vivo, though activating the Akt/FOXO3a pathway. Curr Cancer Drug Targets 16:455–465

Luo S, Lan T, Liao W et al (2012) Genistein inhibits Abeta(2)(5)(-)(3)(5) -induced neurotoxicity in PC12 cells via PKC signaling pathway. Neurochem Res 37:2787–2794

Manach C, Williamson G, Morand C et al (2005) Bioavailability and bioefficacy of polyphenols in humans. I. Review of 97 bioavailability studies. Am J Clin Nutr 81:230s–242s

Messina MJ, Persky V, Setchell KDR et al (1994) Soy intake and cancer risk: a review of the in vitro and in vivo data. Nutr Cancer 21:113–131

Micioni di Bonaventura MV, Cecchini C, Vila-Donat P et al (2017) Evaluation of the hypocholesterolemic effect and prebiotic activity of a lentil (*Lens culinaris* Medik) extract. Mol Nutr Food Res 61(11)

Miller AB, Berrino F, Hill M et al (1994) Diet in the aetiology of cancer: a review. Eur J Cancer 30:207–220

Monagas M, Urpi-Sarda M, Sánchez-Patán F et al (2010) Insights into the metabolism and microbial biotransformation of dietary flavan-3-ols and the bioactivity of their metabolites. Food Funct 1:233–253

Multari S, Neacsu M, Scobbie L et al (2016) Nutritional and phytochemical content of high-protein crops. J Agric Food Chem 64:7800–7811

Muthyala RS, Ju YH, Sheng S et al (2004) Equol, a natural estrogenic metabolite from soy isoflavones. Bioorg Med Chem 12:1559–1567

Nayak B, Liu RH, Berrios JD et al (2011) Bioactivity of antioxidants in extruded products prepared from purple potato and dry pea flours. J Agric Food Chem 59:8233–8243

Neuwirt H, Arias MC, Puhr M et al (2008) Oligomeric proanthocyanidin complexes (OPC) exert anti-proliferative and pro-apoptotic effects on prostate cancer cells. Prostate 68:1647–1654

Oakenfull D, Sidhu G (1984) Prevention of dietary hypercholesterolaemia by chickpea saponins and navy beans. Proc Nutr Soc Aust 9:104

Pavese JM, Krishna SN, Bergan RC (2014) Genistein inhibits human prostate cancer cell detachment, invasion, and metastasis. Am J Clin Nutr 100(Suppl 1):431s–436s

Rabadan-Chavez G, Quevedo-Corona L, Garcia AM et al (2016) Cocoa powder, cocoa extract and epicatechin attenuate hypercaloric diet-induced obesity through enhanced beta-oxidation and energy expenditure in white adipose tissue. J Funct Foods 20:54–67

Rahal OM, Simmen RCM (2010) PTEN and p53 cross-regulation induced by soy isoflavone genistein promotes mammary epithelial cell cycle arrest and lobuloalveolar differentiation. Carcinogenesis 31:1491–1500

Rao A, Sung M (1995) Saponins as anticarcinogens. J Nutr 125:717S

Ray SD, Parikh H, Bagchi D (2005) Proanthocyanidin exposure to B6C3F1 mice significantly attenuates dimethylnitrosamine-induced liver tumor induction and mortality by differentially modulating programmed and unprogrammed cell deaths. Mutat Res 579:81–106

Ridout C, Wharf S, Price K et al (1988) UK mean daily intakes of saponins—intestine-permeabilizing factors in legumes. Food Sci Nutr 42:111–116

Rodriguez de Sotillo DV, Hadley M (2002) Chlorogenic acid modifies plasma and liver concentrations of: cholesterol, triacylglycerol, and minerals in (fa/fa) Zucker rats. J Nutr Biochem 13:717–726

Ruiz RG, Price KR, Arthur AE et al (1996) Effect of soaking and cooking on the saponin content and composition of chickpeas (*Cicer arietinum*) and lentils (*Lens culinaris*). J Agric Food Chem 44:1526–1530

Sautier C, Doucet C, Flament C et al (1979) Effects of soy protein and saponins on serum, tissue and feces steroids in rat. Atherosclerosis 34:233–241

Sergent T, Vanderstraeten J, Winand J et al (2012) Phenolic compounds and plant extracts as potential natural anti-obesity substances. Food Chem 135:68–73

Setchell KDR, Cole SJ (2006) Method of defining equol-producer status and its frequency among vegetarians. J Nutr 136:2188–2193

Shilpi A, Parbin S, Sengupta D et al (2015) Mechanisms of DNA methyltransferase-inhibitor interactions: procyanidin B2 shows new promise for therapeutic intervention of cancer. Chem Biol Interact 233:122–138

Si HW, Fu Z, Babu PVA et al (2011) Dietary epicatechin promotes survival of obese diabetic mice and *Drosophila melanogaster*. J Nutr 141:1095–1100

Sidhu G, Oakenfull D (1986) A mechanism for the hypocholesterolaemic activity of saponins. Br J Nutr 55:643–649

Singletary KW, Meline B (2001) Effect of grape seed proanthocyanidins on colon aberrant crypts and breast tumors in a rat dual-organ tumor model. Nutr Cancer 39:252–258

Sreerama YN, Takahashi Y, Yamaki K (2012) Phenolic antioxidants in some vigna species of legumes and their distinct inhibitory effects on α-glucosidase and pancreatic lipase activities. J Food Sci 77:C927–C933

Tominaga SE (1999) The research group for population-based cancer registration in Japan: cancer incidence in Japan. Cancer mortality and morbidity statistics Japan and the World-1999. Japan Scientific Societies Press, pp 83–144. Retrieved from http://ci.nii.ac.jp/naid/10013440727/en/

Tsunoda N, Pomeroy S, Nestel P (2002) Absorption in humans of isoflavones from soy and red clover is similar. J Nutr 132:2199–2201

van Dijk AE, Olthof MR, Meeuse JC et al (2009) Acute effects of decaffeinated coffee and the major coffee components chlorogenic acid and trigonelline on glucose tolerance. Diabetes Care 32:1023–1025

Verma AK, Johnson JA, Gould MN et al (1988) Inhibition of 7,12-dimethylbenz(a)anthracene- and N-nitrosomethylurea-induced rat mammary cancer by dietary flavonol quercetin. Cancer Res 48:5754–5758

Wang YH, Yang XL, Wang L et al (2010) Effects of proanthocyanidins from grape seed on treatment of recurrent ulcerative colitis in rats. Can J Physiol Pharmacol 88(9):888–898

Wiese S, Esatbeyoglu T, Winterhalter P et al (2015) Comparative biokinetics and metabolism of pure monomeric, dimeric, and polymeric flavan-3-ols: a randomized cross-over study in humans. Mol Nutr Food Res 59:610–621

Willett W, Manson J, Liu SM (2002) Glycemic index, glycemic load, and risk of type 2 diabetes. Am J Clin Nutr 76:274s–280s

Williams AR, Klaver EJ, Laan LC et al (2017) Co-operative suppression of inflammatory responses in human dendritic cells by plant proanthocyanidins and products from the parasitic nematode Trichuris suis. Immunology 150:312–328

Wu WY, Wu YY, Huang H et al (2015a) Biochanin A attenuates LPS-induced pro-inflammatory responses and inhibits the activation of the MAPK pathway in BV2 microglial cells. Int J Mol Med 35:391–398

Wu XY, Xu H, Wu ZF et al (2015b) Formononetin, a novel FGFR2 inhibitor, potently inhibits angiogenesis and tumor growth in preclinical models. Oncotarget 6:44563–44578

Xie Q, Bai Q, Zou LY et al (2014) Genistein inhibits DNA methylation and increases expression of tumor suppressor genes in human breast cancer cells. Genes Chromosom Cancer 53:422–431

Xie Y, Huang S, Su Y (2016) Dietary flavonols intake and risk of esophageal and gastric cancer: a meta-analysis of epidemiological studies. Nutrients 8:91

Xu B, Chang S (2007) A comparative study on phenolic profiles and antioxidant activities of legumes as affected by extraction solvents. J Food Sci 72:S159–S166

Xu B, Chang SKC (2009) Total phenolic, phenolic acid, anthocyanin, flavan-3-ol, and flavonol profiles and antioxidant properties of pinto and black beans (*Phaseolus vulgaris L.*) as affected by thermal processing. J Agric Food Chem 57:4754–4764

Yang H, Xiao L, Yuan Y et al (2014) Procyanidin B2 inhibits NLRP3 inflammasome activation in human vascular endothelial cells. Biochem Pharmacol 92:599–606

Zhang B, Deng Z, Ramdath DD et al (2015) Phenolic profiles of 20 Canadian lentil cultivars and their contribution to antioxidant activity and inhibitory effects on α-glucosidase and pancreatic lipase. Food Chem 172(Supplement C):862–872

Zhang J, Huang YZ, Shao HY et al (2017) Grape seed procyanidin B2 inhibits adipogenesis of 3T3-L1 cells by targeting peroxisome proliferator-activated receptor gamma with miR-483-5p involved mechanism. Biomed Pharmacother 86:292–296

# Chapter 9
# Pulse Processing and Utilization of Pulse Ingredients in Foods

Linda Malcolmson and Jeeyup (Jay) Han

**Abstract** Pulses are a good source of protein and dietary fiber and are rich in vitamins and minerals. Inclusion of pulses in the diet has been shown to be an effective dietary strategy for reducing risk factors for cardiovascular disease and diabetes. Although cooked pulses are consumed in many regions of the world, factors including their long cooking times, the presence of anti-nutritional compounds, and the flatulence associated with their consumption have limited their use but these factors can be minimized through processing. A number of different processing techniques can be applied to pulses including dehulling, splitting, canning, fermentation, germination, roasting, puffing, extrusion, micronization, flour milling, and fractionation. The diverse composition and functionality of processed pulses, pulse flours and pulse fractions provide valuable ingredients for food manufacturers.

**Keywords** Pulses · Dehulling · Fermentation · Extrusion · Micronization · Fractionation · Pulse composition · Pulse flour · Protein concentrate · Hull fiber

## 9.1 Introduction

With global demand for protein increasing, and the high cost and inefficiency in providing protein from animal sources, there is growing interest in protein from plant sources. In particular, greater attention has been directed toward meeting protein needs using pulses alone and in combination with cereals. In addition, their high dietary fiber content and substantial levels of vitamins and minerals make pulses ideal food ingredients. Although cooked pulses have been part of the diet in many regions of the world, several factors have limited their consumption, including their long cooking times, the presence of anti-nutritional compounds, and the

L. Malcolmson (✉)
LM FoodTech Solutions, Winnipeg, MB, Canada

J. (Jay) Han
Food Processing Development Centre, Alberta Agriculture and Forestry, Leduc, AB, Canada
e-mail: jay.han@gov.ab.ca

© Springer Nature Switzerland AG 2019
W. J. Dahl (ed.), *Health Benefits of Pulses*,
https://doi.org/10.1007/978-3-030-12763-3_9

flatulence associated with their consumption. Fortunately, these factors can be minimized through processing.

Pulses contain several anti-nutritional compounds including phytate, enzyme inhibitors (trypsin inhibitors, chymo-trypsin inhibitors, α-amylase inhibitors), polyphenolics (including tannins), lectins, and saponins (Patterson et al. 2017). Although some anti-nutrients have potential benefits for human health (Campos-Vega et al. 2010), compounds such as saponin, phytate, polyphenols, and protease inhibitors can affect the nutritional quality of pulses (Hall et al. 2017). Many of these compounds have been shown to decrease the absorption and digestion of nutrients (Silva-Cristobal et al. 2010). For example, tannins are known to reduce protein digestibility (Hall et al. 2017). Traditional processing methods including soaking, dehulling, boiling, germination and fermentation are effective in reducing levels of anti-nutrients (Patterson et al. 2017). More recent processing techniques include extrusion and micronization show mixed results for reducing anti-nutrients (Patterson et al. 2017) but in the case of micronization, cooking is still required prior to consumption which will reduce anti-nutrient levels. Pulse flours and fractions have also been reported to lower levels of anti-nutrients (Hajos and Osagie 2004).

Pulses can undergo a number of different primary and secondary processing techniques such as dehulling, splitting, canning, fermentation, germination, roasting, puffing, extrusion, micronization, flour milling, and fractionation all of which result in very different pulse products that may require additional processing prior to consumption.

## 9.2  Processing of Pulses

### 9.2.1  Dehulling and Splitting

Dried pulses can be consumed as whole seed or can undergo decortication (dehulling) to remove the seed coat, the purpose of which is mainly to improve digestibility (Siegel and Fawcett 1976), and to reduce cooking time. Both wet and dry methods for decortication can be used (Fig. 9.1). In the wet method, the main objective is to soften the seed coat or hull to ease removal and to eliminate any adherence between the seed coat and the underlying cotyledons. Dehulled seed can then be further processed to split the cotyledons to obtain a product that takes less time to cook. Green and yellow peas, red lentil, and desi chickpea, among others, are commonly processed into splits.

Most pulses, with the exception of split seed and whole lentil, are soaked prior to cooking to hydrate and soften the seeds, thereby reducing the cooking time. Soaking also reduces levels of anti-nutritional compounds such as trypsin inhibitors (Gomes et al. 1979; Wang et al. 2003) and phytic acid (Vidal-Valverde et al. 1994). The soaking step involves hydration to a moisture content of 45–55%. This ensures uniform expansion of the seed coat and cotyledon, as well as cellular hydration to aid in heat transfer and subsequent softening of the seed. The traditional method

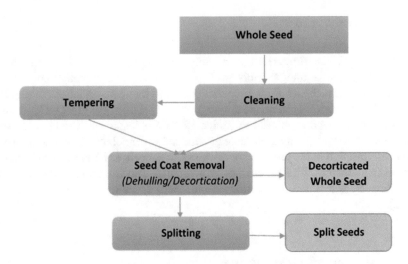

**Fig. 9.1** Schematic diagram of the dehulling and splitting process

involves soaking pulses overnight (8–12 h) in cold water. High temperature soaking can be used to accelerate hydration. Soaking in salt or alkali solutions such as sodium carbonate, sodium bicarbonate and tri-sodium phosphate also can be used, but these treatments may destroy important nutrients.

Cooking in boiling water or pressure cooking are the most common methods used to cook pulses. Cooking results in softening of the cotyledon, thereby increasing palatability as well as inactivating anti-nutritional compounds such as trypsin inhibitors, phytic acid, tannins (Hefnawy 2011; Wang et al. 2003, 2009), and hemagglutinins (Bressani and Elias 1977). Wang et al. (2010) also reported a reduction in oligosaccharide (raffinose, stachyose and verbascose) contents in cooked beans compared to raw beans. Raffinose-family oligosaccharides are thought to be the main contributors to flatulence associated with consuming pulses.

## 9.2.2 Canning

Canning is the most common method of processing pulses, particularly in developed countries. Dried seed is first washed in cold water, drained, and soaked in water for a pre-determined period of time. The soaked seed is drained and a measured amount of seed is placed in each can to which a liquid is added (water, brine or thin sauce). The cans are then vacuum sealed and placed in a retort for processing under pressure to achieve commercial sterility. It is widely recognized that losses of water-soluble vitamins occur during the soaking and canning steps, especially if the liquid in which the pulses are cooked is not consumed. Miller et al. (1973) reported that as much as 50% of the thiamine can be lost during canning. However, it should be pointed out that the elimination or reduction of anti-nutritional compounds during the canning process offsets the loss of vitamins.

### 9.2.3   Fermentation

Fermentation is the process of converting carbohydrates into alcohol or acids through the action of microorganisms. The main benefit of fermenting pulses is an increase in protein digestibility. Enzymes produced by microorganisms during fermentation break down protein into amino acids and peptides and other water soluble products of protein decomposition (Ebine 1972). Robinson and Kao (1974) found that levels of reducing sugars, soluble protein and water-soluble vitamins increased after fermentation in the preparation of chickpea tempeh, a fermented product consumed in Indonesia. The process of fermentation also inactivates anti-nutrients, including trypsin inhibitors, hemagglutinins and saponins (Liener 1962; Ebine 1972).

### 9.2.4   Germination/Sprouting

The germination process involves soaking whole seed for 12 to 24 h in water, after which the soaked seed is allowed to germinate for up to 48 h or until sprouts of 1–2 cm or up to 6 cm in length appear, depending on the desired end-product. Sprouted seed is eaten raw or after cooking. Germination of pulses has been shown to reduce levels of stachyose and raffinose (Snauwaert and Markakis 1976), phytic acid (Reddy et al. 1978; Vidal-Valverde et al. 1994; Devi et al. 2015) and trypsin inhibitors (Gupta and Wagle 1980; Devi et al. 2015) and to increase levels of protein and vitamins (Salunkhe 1985; Devi et al. 2015; Bellaio et al. 2013). Increases in in-vitro protein digestibility and bioavailability of minerals (Jood and Kapoor 1997; Hemalatha et al. 2007) also have been reported.

### 9.2.5   Roasting

Roasting or toasting of pulses involves the exposure of seed to dry heat using temperatures of 150–200 °C. Roasted seeds are often eaten as a snack. Roasting improves flavor and alters the texture of the seed. It also inactivates some of the anti-nutritional compounds found in raw pulses (Jain et al. 2009).

### 9.2.6   Puffing

Pulses may be puffed by subjecting soaked seed to high temperatures (~250 °C) for a short time, approximately 15–25 s (Siegel and Fawcett 1976). Chickpea and pea are the most commonly used pulses for puffing and are eaten in combination with cereals or as a snack.

## 9.2.7  Extrusion

Extrusion cooking is a well-established commercial process used in the production of breakfast cereals and snack foods. The process involves using continuous high pressure, high temperature cooking. The thermomechanical action brings about gelatinization of starches, denaturation of proteins, inactivation of enzymes, microorganisms and anti-nutritional compounds. Research done on the extrusion of pulse flours and high starch fractions, either at 100% or as an inclusion with cereals, has shown good extrusion properties and the production of healthy snack alternatives (Gujska and Khan 1990, 2002; Borejszo and Khan 1992; Balandran-Quintana et al. 1998; Anton et al. 2008a, 2009; Lazou et al. 2010; Hood-Niefer and Tyler 2010; Kelkar et al. 2012; Frohlich et al. 2014; Simons et al. 2015).

## 9.2.8  Micronization

Micronization employs high intensity infrared radiation to achieve rapid internal heating and a rise in water vapour pressure. The process can be described as a 'short time, high temperature' cooking process. Grains, including pulses, are heated in a matter of seconds, without a significant loss of moisture.

When pulses containing sufficient moisture are subjected to micronization, a number of beneficial changes occur including a decrease in trypsin inhibitor (Fasina et al. 2001) and phytic acid (Arntfield et al. 2001) contents, a decrease in protein solubility, and an increase in starch gelatinization which contributes to a reduction in cooking time and an end product that is softer in texture (Arntfield et al. 1997, 2001; Bellido et al. 2006). The partial gelatinization of starch also improves starch digestibility and palatability without significantly affecting other nutrients present (Deepa and Hebbar 2016). Micronization also reduces microbial counts and inactivates enzymes responsible for quality degradation during storage, thereby increasing shelf life.

## 9.2.9  Flour Milling

The milling of pulse flours involves grinding whole or dehulled seeds or splits into small particles. To obtain flour of uniform particle size, ground particles may be passed through one or more screens. The grinding and screening processes may be done separately or may be performed simultaneously in an automated mill such as an impact, knife or roller mill. The properties of the resulting flour depend on whether the seed coat was removed prior to milling or milled separately and added back to the flour. Wholemeal flours have higher fiber contents compared to flours made from dehulled seed, which will affect flour functionality and processing characteristics.

Research has shown that the milling process employed affects the particle size distribution of the flour, along with other properties such as starch damage, pasting properties and water holding capacity (Maskus et al. 2016). Borsuk et al. (2012) and Zucco et al. (2011) found that the particle size of pulse flours significantly influenced the final quality of pita bread and cookies, respectively. In addition, pretreating of pulses prior to milling using infrared heating (Fasina et al. 2001), cooking or roasting (Ma et al. 2011) has also been shown to alter flour functionality.

### 9.2.10  Fractionation

Pulses can be fractionated using wet or dry processes to obtain protein and starch concentrates and isolates, and a fiber fraction as a by-product of the process. By far, the most dominant pulse fractions commercially available are extracted from yellow peas. However, in recent years, other pulses have been commercially fractionated, including lupins, faba beans, mung beans, lentils, chickpeas, cowpeas, great northern beans, lima beans, and navy beans, primarily to obtain the protein fraction.

### 9.2.11  Dry Fractionation

For the dry fractionation process, finely ground, dehulled pulse flour is separated into fractions based on differences in the size and density of particles using a stream of air (Tyler 1984). In commercial operations, dry fractionation uses a combination of impact milling, e.g. pin milling and air classification, which can be repeated to achieve a high recovery rate of the protein fraction (Fig. 9.2). Efficiency of milling and air classification of pulses varies widely based on differences in structural hardness and thickness of seeds and cell walls as well as binding strength between protein bodies and starch granules (Tyler 1984).

The separation principle behind dry fractionation is based on the widely held knowledge that protein bodies are smaller and lighter and have a lower density compared to starch granules. Thus, the fraction with the lower density is high in protein content and referred to as either a "protein concentrate" or a "protein-rich fraction". This fraction contains 50–60% protein. On the other hand, the fraction with the higher density is high in starch content and referred to as either a "starch concentrate" or a "starch-rich fraction" and contains 70–80% starch and 15–20% protein (Youngs 1975; Vose et al. 1976; Han and Khan 1990). This terminology for the fractions is used in the industry; however, no official/scientific definitions have been established. Protein concentrates are used in both the food and pet food industries, whereas starch concentrates have been used mainly in animal feed or in the pet food industry because of their relatively high protein content (15–20%) and low price. Although the utilization of pulse starches in food products has been limited, their functional properties, especially their physical and thermal characteristics,

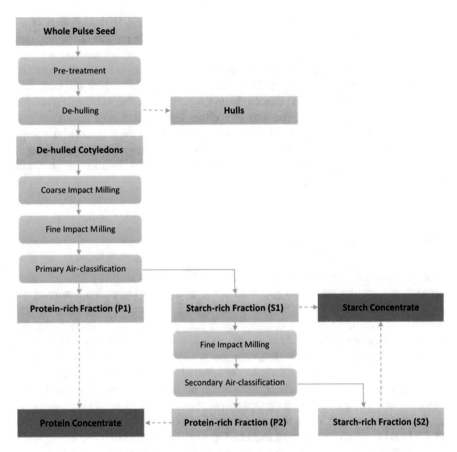

**Fig. 9.2** Schematic diagram of dry fractionation of pulse protein and starch concentrates

have been identified and potential applications in food products have been studied. With the growing demand for vegetable protein, the starch concentrate could be used as feedstock for the extraction of additional protein or to obtain a purified starch product via a wet extraction process.

Tyler et al. (1981) compared the protein content of fractions prepared from different pulses (cowpea, great northern bean, lima bean, mung bean, navy bean, lentil, faba bean and field pea) using flours produced by pin milling followed by air classification. Faba bean (63.8–75.1%) and lima bean (43.4–49.6%) were found to have the highest and lowest levels of protein in the protein-rich fractions. Differences in minor constituents (fiber, resistant starch, lipid, and ash) levels will also vary depending on the fraction, pulse type, and the processing conditions employed. For example, studies have reported a wide range of levels for minor constituents in dry fractionated protein fractions with values for fiber of 0.85% (dehulled great northern bean) to 2.1% (dehulled navy bean), for lipid of 0.97% (great northern bean) to 3.49% (small white bean), and for ash of 1.60% (navy bean) to 7.8% (great northern bean)

(Satterlee et al. 1975; Kon et al. 1977; Sosulski and Youngs 1979; Aguilera et al. 1982; Gujska and Khan 1991; Rui et al. 2011). Difference in protein, starch, and minor constituent levels in the fractions will affect functionality including solubility, water binding capacity, emulsifying and foaming capacity and stability, thickening and gel-forming capacities, and freeze-thaw syneresis. This in turn will influence the overall quality of the food prepared from the fraction. Understanding the unique functional properties of the fractions as well as their performance under various processing conditions (e.g. pH, temperature) will allow for the successful development of food products prepared from fractions (Farooq and Boye 2011; Azarphazhooh and Boye 2013). A more detailed review on pulse protein functionality can be found in Singhal et al. (2016).

## 9.2.12 Wet Fractionation

The wet fractionation process is a more complex process than dry fractionation. Several wet protein extraction processes have been used in the food industry to separate higher purity fractions from a heterogeneous mixture. Depending on the material of interest to isolate, different extraction processes, or a combination of processes, can be used. One of the most widely used wet extraction processes is alkaline extraction of protein followed by isoelectric precipitation and drying (Fig. 9.3). The alkaline extraction process is based on protein solubility as a function of the environmental conditions employed during the process, principally pH, but also ionic strength and temperature (Boye et al. 2010a). In the wet extraction of pulses, the process begins by dispersing dehulled pulse flour in water using a ratio of 1:5 to 1:15, w/v, flour to water, followed by adjusting the pH of the slurry to 8–11 using sodium hydroxide. The slurrification step can also be achieved by wet milling of pre-soaked dehulled seeds in water. The slurry is then stirred for 1–4 h at any of a variety of temperatures (10–50 °C) to maximize the solubilisation of protein. In general, protein solubility/recovery increases with temperature, hence extraction at a lower temperature requires a longer extraction time. For example, for some defatted flours, a low temperature extraction is run overnight (10–16 h). The processing conditions for protein extraction vary depending on the type of protein or pulse. The solubilized protein is then separated from insoluble materials (starch, cell wall fiber) by a combination of screening, centrifugation, filtration, and/or hydrocyclone separation. The pH of the protein extract is adjusted to the isoelectric point (pH 4–5) using dilute acid. At the isoelectric pH, much of the solubilised protein will precipitate and is recovered by centrifugation or filtration. Finally, the pH of the recovered protein is adjusted to near neutrality and the protein product is spray dried. A variety of modifications and adjustments have been made to the alkaline extraction process, depending on the desired properties of the final product (Chew et al. 2003; Papalamprou et al. 2009). A number of alternative protein extraction and recovery processes also have been developed, including water, salt and acid extraction, and recovery of protein by ultrafiltration. Wet fractionation has been reviewed by Hoover et al. (2010), Naguleswaran and Vasanthan (2010), and Tiwari and Singh (2012).

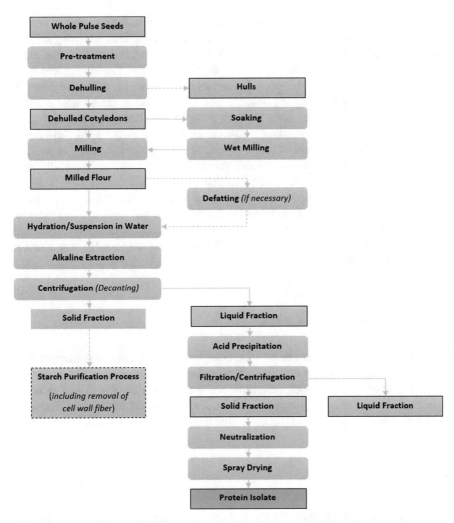

**Fig. 9.3** Schematic diagram of a wet extraction process for pulse protein and starch isolates using isoelectric precipitation

The starch and protein fractions obtained from a wet extraction process are of higher purity compared to those obtained from a dry fractionation process. The protein content of the protein fraction is usually in the range of 70–89% and is referred to as a "protein isolate." The starch fraction or "starch isolate", contains 1–15% protein and 75–95% starch depending on the particular extraction process employed. Further concentration of the protein content can be obtained using a secondary process, such as aqueous-alcohol washing, acid washing, hot water extraction, or enzyme treatment (Han and Hamaker 2002). Comparison of protein levels achieved in protein isolates prepared from different pulses is difficult since secondary processing methods vary. A review has been published by Boye et al. (2010b) which reports published values for protein levels achieved using different processing conditions and pulse types. The secondary processes can also be used to modify protein and starch functionality of the extracted fractions including solubility, water and fat binding capacities, emulsifying, foaming, and gelling properties, thickening and flavour binding (Ratnayake et al. 2002; Boye et al. 2010b; Roy et al. 2010; Sun and Arntfield 2010). Protein functional properties are affected by protein structure and formation, hydrophobicity and hydrophilicity, amino acid composition and processing conditions used to produce the food products. Like concentrates, isolates contain minor constituents such as fiber, lipid, non-starch carbohydrates, minerals, and vitamins which can influence functionality. In terms of flavor and color, protein and starch isolates are lighter in color and generally have less flavor than protein and starch concentrates.

In addition to protein and starch isolates, the wet extraction processes produces a by-product that is rich in fiber. This fiber fraction is derived from cell wall material (Guillon and Champ 2002) and is correctly characterized as inner cotyledon cell wall fiber. It is composed mainly of soluble fiber in contrast to hull fiber, which is primarily insoluble fiber.

## 9.3    Composition of Pulses

Pulses are excellent sources of protein, complex carbohydrates (including dietary fiber), vitamins and minerals. Variability in the chemical composition of pulses occurs among market classes, genotypes within a market class, and as a result of geographic location and growing conditions. A more detailed review on the composition and nutritional value of pulses has recently been published (Hall et al. 2017).

### 9.3.1    Protein

Pulses have twice the amount of protein as cereals, with a protein content of 22–26% for peas, beans, lentils and chickpeas (Wang and Daun 2004, 2006; USDA 2012), and higher levels associated with faba beans (27–34%; Duc 1997, Hacıseferoğulları et al. 2003) and lupins (33–47%: Erbas et al. 2005; Rumiyati et al. 2012). This is in contrast to cereal grains, with protein levels of 9–15% for wheat, 7–13% for barley and 2–5% for rice. Pulse proteins are low in the sulphur containing amino acids cysteine and methionine, but high in lysine. Cereal grains, conversely, are low in lysine. Thus, including pulses with cereals will greatly enhance protein quality. In contrast to wheat flour, the major proteins found in pulses are globulins and albumins (Boye et al. 2010b) which limits the full replacement of wheat flour with pulse flours and fractions in products where gluten development is required. Other minor proteins in pulses include prolamins and glutelins (Gupta and Dhillon 1993; Saharan and Khetarpaul 1994).

Although proteins in pulses have been found to be allergenic, allergic reactions to pulses are limited and have been confined mostly to Europe, Asia and the Mediterranean (San Ireneo et al. 2000), likely due to their higher consumption in these populations (Boye et al. 2010b). Severe anaphylaxis to pulses is infrequent (San Ireneo et al. 2000) which may explain why pulses are not classified as major allergens with the exception of lupins which is a declared allergen in Australia and the EU.

Functional properties of food proteins that are important in food processing include solubility, water and fat binding capacities, foaming and emulsifying properties, thickening and gel formation (Boye et al. 2010b). These properties will influence the texture and sensory characteristics of final products. In general, pulse flours and protein fractions exhibit good protein functionality, although their functional properties will vary depending on pulse type and the method and conditions used for milling and/or fractionation.

## 9.3.2 Starch

Starch is the major storage polysaccharide in pulses and ranges in concentration from 35% to 60%. Pulse starch is composed mainly of amylose and amylopectin and contains a higher proportion of amylose (24–65%) compared to starches from cereals and tubers. The amylose content of pulse starches is influenced by market class and genotype within a market class, with values of 33–44% for pea (Ratnayake et al. 2001; Sangdhu and Lim 2008), 22–32% for lentil (Hoover and Ratnayake 2002; Sangdhu and Lim 2008), 21–34% for chickpea (Hoover and Ratnayake 2002; Hughes et al. 2009), 23–38% for black bean (Hoover and Ratnayake 2002, Sangdhu and Lim 2008) and 26% for navy bean (Hoover and Ratnayake 2002), as determined by an iodine-binding method. The size and shape of pulse starch granules varies depending on genotype. Granules range in size from 5 to 104 μm and are round, spherical or oval in shape (Hoover et al. 1997, 2010). Pulse starch pastes are generally more viscous and have more resistance to rupture under shear stress compared to cereal starches. Both peak viscosity and breakdown viscosity of pulse starches are dependent on amylose content, granule size distribution, and amylopectin structure, which vary with market class.

## 9.3.3 Fiber

Pulses are a good source of dietary fiber, both soluble and insoluble (Table 9.1). Processing can alter dietary fiber content, especially its composition and physiological properties. Cooking significantly decreases the total dietary fiber content of pulses, but also increases the resistant starch content (Kutoš et al. 2003). The increase in resistant starch most likely results from the retrogradation of starch after

**Table 9.1** Dietary fiber content of dried pulses

| Market class | Dietary fiber | | | Reference |
| --- | --- | --- | --- | --- |
| | Total | Insoluble | Soluble | |
| Pea | 14–26 | 11.3 | 8.7 | Dalgetty and Baik (2003) |
| Lentil | 18–20 | 11.4 | 6.9 | Dalgetty and Baik (2003) |
| Chickpea | 18–22 | 10.0 | 8.4 | Dalgetty and Baik (2003) |
| Pinto bean | 23.3 | 19.8 | 3.5 | Kutos et al. (2003) |
| Small red bean | 21.6 | 18.0 | 3.6 | Wang et al. (2010) |
| Red kidney bean | 20.0 | 15.0 | 5.0 | Wang et al. (2010) |
| Common beans | – | 20.0–22.6 | 2.4–2.6 | De Almeida Costa et al. (2006) |

gelatinization. Many physicochemical and functional properties of pulse flours and ingredients, such as water-binding capacity, bulk density, viscosity, gelling properties, and fermentability, can be attributed to their fiber content.

## 9.4 Use of Pulse Ingredients in Foods

Although the vast majority of pulses are sold as whole or split dried seeds, there is a tremendous opportunity to expand the use of pulses in processed foods using pulse flours and fractions. Fig. 9.4 provides a schematic of the possible uses of pea ingredients in foods. Similar possibilities exist for other pulses.

Extensive research has been undertaken to investigate the use of pulse flours and fractions in foods (Table 9.2). Pulse flours have been successfully used to either partially replace wheat flour or gluten-free starches and flours to enhance nutrient content and/or improve functionality in a range of food products. In general, pulse flours can be substituted for wheat flour at levels ranging between 10% and 30% with minimal impact on end quality and processing conditions. The exact level of substitution is dependent on the product and the requirement for gluten to give the desired structure to the product. In terms of gluten-free applications, pulse flours can be substituted for starches and flours at similar levels depending on the formulation and end product. Pulse flours can affect the flavour of the finished product with pea and lentil flours have a greater impact on flavour than chickpea and bean flours. Color of the final product can also be affected depending on the pulse flour used and the product which the flour is being added to. Besides pulse type and the possible use of pulse flour blends, consideration should be given to the flour particle size to achieve optimal flour performance in the product. Furthermore, the use of heat treated or pre-cooked pulse flours, primarily done to reduce flavour issues, can significantly alter flour functionality which will in turn affect final product quality.

Protein fractions are mainly added to foods to boost protein content to meet protein claims although researchers have shown that pea protein fractions could be successfully used to replace eggs in a variety of baked products and pastas (Northern Pulse Growers n.d.). Protein concentrates are lower in protein (50–60%) than

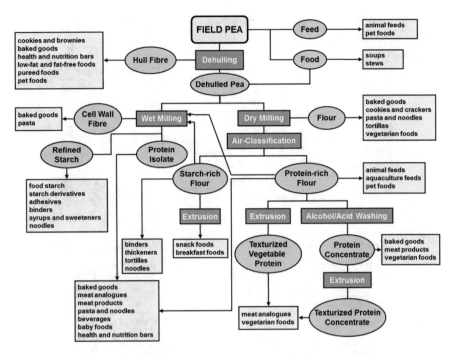

**Fig. 9.4** Utilization of pea ingredients in food applications (Han and Tyler 2010)

isolates (70–89%) and will differ in functionality due to differences in the processing methods used to obtain the fraction and the level of other constituents (starch, resistant starch, fiber, etc.) in the fraction. Pulse starch fractions have few commercial applications due to their restricted swelling power, poor granule dispersibility, high gelatinization transition temperatures, high extent of water exudation (syneresis) and resistance to enzyme hydrolysis (Hoover et al. 2010). Research has shown however, that native pea starch can replace modified corn starch in coatings for French fries, mozzarella sticks and onion rings with minimal impact on processing and product quality (Pulse Canada n.d.).

Both pea hull and inner cell wall fiber fractions can be added to conventional and gluten free formulations to increase fiber content of foods and improve functional properties of food formulations. Levels of inclusion are generally around 5%. Since the two fractions differ in composition, with hull fiber containing mainly insoluble fiber and cell wall fiber containing mainly soluble fiber they have different functional properties in foods. Both pea hull fiber and cell wall fiber were shown to improve cooking yields of ground beef and pork patties but did not impact cooking yields of chicken patties (Manitoba Food Development Centre 2015). Pea cell wall fiber have also been shown to have good fat retaining and texture modifying properties in low and high fat beef patties (Anderson and Berry 2000, 2001a, b).

**Table 9.2** Summary of food applications using pulse flours and fractions

| Objective | Food product | Pulse ingredient | References |
|---|---|---|---|
| Fiber enrichment | | | |
| | Muffins | Bean hull fiber | Daubenmire et al. (1993) |
| | Cookies | Bean hull fiber | DeFouw et al. (1982a) |
| | | Bean hull fiber | Jeltema et al. (1983) |
| | | Pea hull fiber | Piteira et al. (2006) |
| | Cake | Bean hull fiber | DeFouw et al. (1982b) |
| | Bread | Pea, lentil, chickpea hull fibers and cell wall fibers | Dalgetty and Baik (2006) |
| | | | Rosell et al. (2006) |
| | | Pea cell wall fiber | Collar et al. (2006, 2007) |
| | | Pea hull fiber | Sosulski and Wu (1988) |
| | | | Gómez et al. (2003) |
| | | | Wang et al. (2002) |
| | Bagels and tortillas | Pea hull fiber, pea cell wall fiber | Malcolmson et al. (2013) |
| | Pasta | Pea cell wall fiber | Edwards et al. (1995) |
| | | Pea hull fiber | Tudorica et al. (2002) |
| Nutrient fortification/enhancement | | | |
| | Cake | Chickpea flour | Gómez et al. (2008) |
| | Cookies | Lentil, bean flours | Zucco et al. (2011) |
| | Tortillas | Bean flour | Anton et al. (2008b) |
| | | Bean, chickpea, pea, lentil flours | Malcolmson et al. (2013) |
| | Pita bread | Chickpea, pea, lentil flours | Malcolmson et al. (2013) |
| | | Lentil, bean flours | Borsuk et al. (2012) |
| | Bread | Chickpea flour | Utrilla-Coello et al. (2007) |
| | Crackers | Lentil flour | Malcolmson et al. (2013) |
| | Quick breads, muffins | Bean flour | Alani et al. (1989), Dryer et al. (1982), and Cady et al. (1987) |
| | Doughnuts | Bean flour | Spink et al. (1984) |
| | Pasta | Bean, lentil flours | Bahnassey et al. (1986) |
| | | Chickpea, lentil, pea flours | Zhao et al. (2005) |
| | Extruded snacks | Pea, lentil, chickpea flours, pea hull fiber | Frohlich et al. (2014) |
| | | | Anton et al. (2008a, 2009) |
| | | Bean flour | Balandran-Quintana et al. (1998) |
| | | | Simons et al. (2015) |
| | | | Kelkar et al. (2012) |
| | | | Hood-Niefer and Tyler (2010) |
| | | Pea flour | Lazou et al. (2010) |
| | | Lentil flour | Gujska and Khan (1990 and 2002) |
| | | High starch bean fractions | Borejszo and Khan (1992) |
| | Beverages | Chickpea, lentil flours, pea hull fiber, pea protein | Zare et al. (2015) |
| | Salad dressings | Chickpea, lentil, pea flours | Ma et al. (2016a, b) |
| | Yogurt | Lentil flour | Zare et al. (2011) |

(continued)

**Table 9.2** (continued)

| Objective | Food product | Pulse ingredient | References |
|---|---|---|---|
| Fat binding | | | |
| | High-fat beef patties | Pea cell wall fiber | Anderson and Berry (2001a, b) |
| Texture modification | | | |
| | Low-fat bologna | Chickpea flour | Sanjeewa et al. (2010) |
| | Low-fat beef patties | Pea flour, fiber, starch | Pietrasik and Janz (2010) |
| | Low-fat sausages sausages | Pea cell wall fiber | Anderson and Berry (2000) |
| | Meat analog | Pea flour | Kaack and Pedersen (2005) |
| | Low-fat fish sausage | Chickpea flour | Verma et al. (1984) |
| | | Pea protein isolate | Osen et al. (2014) |
| | | Pea cell wall fiber | Cardoso et al. (2008) |
| Gluten-free | | | |
| | Pizza crust | Chickpea, pea, lentil flours | Malcolmson et al. (2013) |
| | Cookies | Pea flour | Malcolmson et al. (2013) |
| | Crackers | Bean flour | Simons and Hall (2018) |
| | Bread | Chickpea, lentil, pea, bean flours, pea protein, starch, fibre | Han et al. (2010) |
| | | Chickpea flour, pea protein isolate | Miñarro et al. (2012) |

## 9.5  Summary

Although pulses have a long history of use, there is growing interest in using pulses and pulse ingredients to meet consumer demand for foods that deliver nutritional benefits. Pulses with their high protein and fiber levels and abundant levels of vitamins and minerals along with their reported health benefits make pulses valuable food ingredients for food manufacturers. A range of pulse types are available, each with their own unique color and flavor profiles which allows for versatility in formulating products. In addition, pulses can undergo various processing techniques including fermentation, germination, roasting, puffing, extrusion, micronization, flour milling and fractionation to produce novel food products and/or ingredients. Research has shown that pulse flours and fractions can be successfully used in a range of foods to fortify nutritional content and to provide enhanced functionality in both wheat based and gluten free applications.

## References

Aguilera JM, Lucas EW, Uebersax MA et al (1982) Development of food ingredients from navy beans (*Phaseolus vulgaris*) by roasting, pin milling, and air classification. J Food Sci 47:1151–1154

Alani SR, Zabik ME, Uebersax MA (1989) Dry roasted pinto bean (*Phaseolus vulgaris*) flour in quick breads. Cereal Chem 66:348–349

Anderson ET, Berry BW (2000) Sensory, shear, and cooking properties of lower-fat beef patties made with inner pea fiber. J Food Sci 65:805–810

Anderson ET, Berry BW (2001a) Identification of nonmeat ingredients for increasing fat holding capacity during heating of ground beef. J Food Qual 24:291–299

Anderson ET, Berry BW (2001b) Effects of inner pea fiber on fat retention and cooking yield in high fat ground beef. Food Res Int 34:689–694

Anton AA, Luciano FB, Maskus H (2008a) Development of Globix: a new bean-based pretzel-like snack. Cereal Foods World 53:70–74

Anton AA, Ross KA, Lukow OM et al (2008b) Influence of added bean flour (*Phaseolus vulgaris L.*) on some physical and nutritional properties of wheat flour tortillas. Food Chem 109:33–41

Anton AA, Fulcher RG, Arntfield AD (2009) Physical and nutritional impact of fortification of corn starch-based extruded snacks with common bean (*Phaseolus vulgaris* L.) flour: effects of bean addition and extrusion cooking. Food Chem 113:989–996

Arntfield SD, Scanlon MG, Malcolmson LJ et al (1997) Effect of tempering and end moisture content on the quality of micronized lentils. Food Res Int 30:371–380

Arntfield SD, Scanlon MG, Malcolmson LJ et al (2001) Reduction in lentil cooking time using micronization: comparison of two micronization temperatures. J Food Sci 66:500–505

Azarphazhooh E, Boye JI (2013) Composition of processed dry beans and pulses. In: Siddiq M, Uebersax MA (eds) Dry beans and pulses: production, processing and nutrition. Wiley-Blackwell, Ames, pp 103–128

Bahnassey Y, Khan K, Harrold R (1986) Fortification of spaghetti with edible legumes. I. Physicochemical, antinutritional, amino acid, and mineral composition. Cereal Chem 63:210–215

Balandran-Quintana RR, Barbosa-Canovas GV, Zazueta-Morales JJ et al (1998) Functional and nutritional properties of extruded whole pinto bean meal (*Phaseolus vulgaris L*). J Food Sci 63:113–116

Bellaio S, Kappeler S, Rosenfeld EZ et al (2013) Partially germinated ingredients for naturally healthy and tasty products. Cereal Foods World 58:55–59

Bellido G, Arntfield SD, Cenkowski S et al (2006) Effects of micronization pretreatments on the physicochemical properties of navy and black beans (*Phaseolus vulgaris* L.). LWT-Food Sci Technol 39:779–787

Borejszo Z, Khan K (1992) Reduction of flatulence-causing sugars by high temperature extrusion of pinto bean high starch fractions. J Food Sci 57:771–777

Borsuk Y, Arntfield S, Lukow OM et al (2012) Incorporation of pulse flours of different particle size in relation to pita bread quality. J Sci Food Agric 92:2055–2061

Boye JI, Aksay S, Roufik S et al (2010a) Comparison of the functional properties of pea, chickpea and lentil protein concentrates processed using ultrafiltration and isoelectric precipitation techniques. Food Res Int 43:537–546

Boye J, Zare F, Pletch A (2010b) Pulse proteins: processing, characterization, functional properties and applications in food and feed. Food Res Int 43:414–431

Bressani R, Elias LG (1977) In: National standards and methods of evaluation for food legume breeders, IDRC, Ottawa p 51

Cady ND, Carter AE, Kayne BE et al (1987) Navy bean flour substitution in a master mix used for muffins and cookies. Cereal Chem 64:193–195

Campos-Vega R, Loarca-Pina G, Oomah BD (2010) Minor components of pulses and their potential impact on human health. Food Res Int 43:461–482

Cardoso C, Mendes R, Nunes ML (2008) Development of a healthy low-fat fish sausage containing dietary fibre. Int J Food Sci Technol 43:276–283

Chew PG, Andrew C, Stuart J (2003) Protein quality and physico-functionality of Australian sweet lupin (*Lupinus angustifolius* cv. *Gungurru*) protein concentrates prepared by isoelectric precipitation or ultrafiltration. Food Chem 83:575–583

Collar C, Santos E, Rosell CM (2006) Significance of dietary fiber on the viscometric pattern of pasted and gelled flour fiber blends. Cereal Chem 83:370–376

Collar C, Santos E, Rosell CM (2007) Assessment of the rheological profile of fibre-enriched bread doughs by response surface methodology. J Food Eng 78:820–826

Dalgetty DD, Baik B-K (2003) Isolation and characterization of cotyledon fibers from peas, lentils and chickpeas. Cereal Chem 80(3):310–315

Dalgetty DD, Baik B-K (2006) Fortification of bread with hulls and cotyledon fibers isolated from peas, lentils and chickpeas. Cereal Chem 83:269–274

Daubenmire SW, Zabik ME, Setser CS (1993) Development of low fat, cholesterol-free, high-fiber muffins. 1. Fiber source and particle size effects on quality characteristics. FAO. Sch Food Serv Res Rev 17:15–20

De Almeida Costa GE, Da Silva Q-MK, Pissini Machado Reis SM et al (2006) Chemical composition, dietary fiber and resistant starch contents of raw and cooked pea, common bean, chickpea and lentil legumes. Food Chem 94:327–330

Deepa C, Hebbar HU (2016) Effect of high-temperature short-time 'micronization' of gains on product quality and cooking characteristics. Food Eng Rev 8:201–203

DeFouw C, Zabik ME, Uebersax MA et al (1982a) Effect of heat treatment and level of navy bean hulls in sugar-snap cookies. Cereal Chem 59:245–248

DeFouw C, Zabik ME, Uebersax MA et al (1982b) Use of unheated and heat treated navy bean hulls as a source of dietary fiber in spice flavored layer cakes. Cereal Chem 59:229–230

Devi CB, Kushwaha A, Kumar A (2015) Sprouting characteristics and associated changes in nutritional composition of cowpea (*Vigna unguiculata*). J Food Sci Technol 52:6821–6827

Dryer SB, Phillips SG, Powell TS et al (1982) Dry roasted navy bean flour incorporation in a quick bread. Cereal Chem 59:319–320

Duc G (1997) Faba bean (*Vicia faba L.*). Field Crop Res 53(1–3):99–109

Ebine H (1972) Fermented soybean foods in Japan. Trop Agric Res Ser 6:217–223

Edwards NM, Biliaderis CG, Dexter JE (1995) Textural characteristics of whole wheat pasta and pasta containing non-starch polysaccharides. J Food Sci 60:1321–1324

Erbas M, Certel M, Uslu MK (2005) Some chemical properties of white lupin seeds (*Lupinus albus L.*). Food Chem 89:341–345

Farooq Z, Boye JI (2011) Novel food and industrial application of pulse flours and fractions. In: Tiwari BK, Gowen A, McKenna B (eds) Pulse foods: processing, quality and nutraceutical applications. Academic, London, pp 103–128

Fasina OO, Tyler RT, Pickard MD et al (2001) Effect of infrared heating on properties of legume seeds. Int J Food Sci Technol 36:79–90

Frohlich P, Boux G, Malcolmson L (2014) Pulse ingredients as healthier options in extruded products. Cereal Foods World 59:120–125

Gomes JC, Koch U, Brunner JR (1979) Isolation of a trypsin inhibitor from navy beans by affinity chromatography. Cereal Chem 56:525–529

Gómez M, Ronda F, Blanco CA et al (2003) Effect of dietary fibre on dough rheology and bread quality. Eur Food Res Technol 216:51–56

Gómez M, Oliete B, Rosell CM et al (2008) Studies on cake quality made of wheat–chickpea flour blends. LWT-Food Sci Technol 41:1701–1709

Guillon F, Champ MM (2002) Carbohydrate fractions of legumes: uses in human nutrition and potential for health. Br J Nutr 88(Suppl 3):S293–S306

Gujska E, Khan K (1990) Effect of temperature on properties of extrudates from high starch fractions of navy, pinto and garbanzo beans. J Food Sci 55:466–469

Gujska E, Khan K (1991) Functional properties of extrudates from high starch fractions of navy and pinto beans and corn meal blended with legume high protein fractions. J Food Sci 56:431–435

Gujska E, Khan K (2002) Effect of extrusion variables on amino acids, available lysine and in vitro protein digestibility of the extrudates from pinto bean (*Phaseolus vulgaris L.*). Pol J Food Nutr Sci 52:39–43

Gupta R, Dhillon S (1993) Characterization of seed storage proteins of lentil (*Lens culinaris M.*). Ann Biol 9:71–78

Gupta K, Wagle DS (1980) Changes in antinutritional factors during germination in *Phaseolus mungoreous*, a cross between *Phaseolus mungo* (M1–1) and *Phaseolus aureus* (T1). J Food Sci 45:394–397

Hacıseferoğulları H, Gezer I, Bahtiyarca YCHO et al (2003) Determination of some chemical and physical properties of Sakız faba bean (*Vicia faba L.* Var. major). J Food Eng 60:475–479

Hajos G, Osagie AU (2004) Technical and biotechnical modifications of antinutritional factors in legumes and oilseeds. Proceedings of 4th International Workshop on Antinutritional Factors in Legume Seeds and Oilseeds, pp 293–305

Hall C, Hillen C, Garden Robinson J (2017) Composition, nutritional value, and health benefits of pulses. Cereal Chem 94:11–31

Han Z, Hamaker BR (2002) Partial leaching of granule-associated proteins from rice starch during alkaline extraction and subsequent gelatinization. Starch-Starke 54:454–460

Han JY, Khan K (1990) Physicochemical studies of pin-milled and air-classified dry edible bean fractions. Cereal Chem 67:384–390

Han JY, Tyler RT (2010) Unpublished data. University of Saskatchewan

Han JY, Janz JAM, Gerlat M (2010) Development of gluten-free cracker snacks using pulse flours and fractions. Food Res Int 43:627–633

Hefnawy TH (2011) Effect of processing methods on nutritional composition and anti-nutritional factors in lentils (*Lens culinaris*). Ann Agric Sci 56:57–61

Hemalatha S, Platel K, Srinivasan K (2007) Influence of germination and fermentation on bioaccessibility of zinc and iron from food grains. Eur J Clin Nutr 61:342–348

Hood-Niefer SD, Tyler RT (2010) Effect of protein, moisture content and barrel temperature on the physicochemical characteristics of pea flour extrudates. Food Res Int 43:659–663

Hoover R, Ratnayake WS (2002) Starch characteristics of black bean, chick pea, lentil, navy bean and pinto bean cultivars grown in Canada. Food Chem 78:489–498

Hoover R, Li YX, Hynes G et al (1997) Physico- chemical characterization of mung bean starch. Food Hydrocoll 11:401–408

Hoover R, Hughes T, Chung HJ et al (2010) Composition, molecular structure, properties, and modification of pulse starches: a review. Food Res Int 43:399–413

Hughes T, Hoover R, Liu Q et al (2009) Composition, morphology, molecular structure, and physicochemical properties of starches from newly released chickpea (*Cicer arietinum* L.) cultivars grown in Canada. Food Res Int 42:627–635

Jain AK, Kumar S, Panwar JDS (2009) Antinutritional factors and their detoxification in pulses-a review. Agric Rev 30:64–70

Jeltema MA, Zabik ME, Thiel LJ (1983) Prediction of cookie quality from dietary fiber components. Cereal Chem 60:227–230

Jood S, Kapoor AC (1997) Improvement in bioavailability of minerals of chickpea and blackgram cultivars through processing and cooking methods. Int J Food Sci Nutr 48:307–312

Kaack K, Pedersen L (2005) Low energy chocolate cake with potato pulp and yellow pea hulls. Eur Food Res Technol 221:367–375

Kelkar S, Siddiq M, Harte JB et al (2012) Use of low-temperature extrusion for reducing phytohemagglutinin activity (PHA) and oligosaccharides in beans (*Phaseolus vulgaris L*) cv. Navy and Pinto. Food Chem 133:1636–1639

Kon S, Sanshuck DW, Jackson R et al (1977) Air classification of bean flour. J Food Process Preserv 1:69–77

Kutoš T, Golob T, Kač M et al (2003) Dietary fibre content of dry and processed beans. Food Chem 80:231–235

Lazou A, Krokida M, Tzia C (2010) Sensory properties and acceptability of corn and lentil extruded puffs. J Sens Stud 25:838–860

Liener IE (1962) Toxic protein from the soybean. II. Physical characterization. Am J Clin Nutr 11:281–286

Ma Z, Boye JI, Simpson BK et al (2011) Thermal processing effects on the functional properties and microstructure of lentil, chickpea, and pea flours. Food Res Int 44:2534–2544

Ma Z, Boye JI, Swallow K et al (2016a) Techno-functional characterization of salad dressing emulsions supplemented with pea, lentil and chickpea flours. J Sci Food Agric 96:837–847

Ma Z, Boye JI, Simpson BK (2016b) Preparation of salad dressing emulsions using lentil, chickpea and pea protein isolates: a response surface methodology study. J Food Qual 39:274–291

Malcolmson L, Boux G, Bellido A-S et al (2013) Use of pulse ingredients to develop healthier baked products. Cereal Foods World 58:27–32

Manitoba Food Development Centre (2015) https://www.manitobapulse.ca/wp-content/uploads/2015/10/Pea-Fibre-Utilization-in-Ground-Poultry-Beef-and-Pork.pdf. Accessed 4 Oct 2018

Maskus H, Bourré L, Fraser S et al (2016) Effects of grinding method on the compositional, physical, and functional properties of whole and split yellow pea flours. Cereal Foods World 61:59–64

Miller CF, Guadagni DG, Kon S (1973) Vitamin retention in bean products: cooked, canned and instant bean powders. J Food Sci 38:493–495

Miñarro B, Albanell E, Aguilar N et al (2012) Effect of legume flours on baking characteristics of gluten-free bread. J Cereal Sci 56:476–481

Naguleswaran S, Vasanthan T (2010) Dry milling of field pea (*Pisum sativum* L.) groats prior to wet fractionation influences the starch yield and purity. Food Chem 118:627–633

Northern Pulse Growers (n.d.) https://northernpulse.com/uploads/resources/658/pea-protein-brochure.pdf. Accessed 4 Oct 2018

Osen R, Toelstede S, Wild F et al (2014) High moisture extrusion cooking of pea protein isolates: raw material characteristics, extruder responses, and texture properties. J Food Eng 127:67–74

Papalamprou EM, Doxastakis GI, Biliaderis CG et al (2009) Influence on preparation methods on physicochemical and gelation properties of chickpea protein isolates. Food Hydrocoll 23:337–343

Patterson CA, Curran J, Der T (2017) Effect of processing on antinutrient compounds in pulses. Cereal Chem 94:2–10

Pietrasik Z, Janz JAM (2010) Utilization of pea flour, starch-rich and fiber-rich fractions in low fat bologna. Food Res Int 43:602–608

Piteira MF, Maia JM, Raymundo A et al (2006) Extensional flow behaviour of natural fiber-filled dough and its relationship with structure and properties. J Non-Newtonian Fluid Mech 137:72–80

Pulse Canada (n.d.) http://www.pulsecanada.com/wp-content/uploads/2017/09/Pulses-in-Batter-and-Breading-Applications.pdf. Accessed 3 Oct 2018

Ratnayake WS, Hoover R, Shahidi F et al (2001) Composition, molecular structure, and physico-chemical properties of starches from four field pea (*Pisum sativum* L.) cultivars. Food Chem 74:189–202

Ratnayake WS, Hoover R, Warkentin T (2002) Pea starch: Composition, structure and properties - a review. Starch-Stärke 54(6):217–234

Reddy NR, Balakrishnan CV, Salunkhe DK (1978) Phytate phosphorus and mineral changes during germination and cooking of black gram (*Phaseolus mungo* L.) seeds. J Food Sci 43:540–542

Robinson RJ, Kao C (1974) Fermented foods from chickpeas, horse beans, and soybeans. Cereal Sci Today 19:397 (Abstract)

Rosell CM, Santos E, Collar C (2006) Mixing properties of fibre enriched wheat bread doughs: a response surface methodology study. Eur Food Res Technol 223:333–340

Roy F, Boye JI, Simpson BK (2010) Bioactive proteins and peptides in pulse crops: Pea, chickpea and lentil. Food Res Int 43(2):432–442

Rui X, Boye JL, Ribereau S et al (2011) Comparative study of the composition and thermal properties of protein isolates prepared from nine *Phaseouls vulgaris* legume varieties. Food Res Int 44:2497–2504

Rumiyati R, James AP, Jayasena V (2012) Effect of germination on the nutritional and protein profile of Australian sweet lupin (*Lupinus angustifolius* L.). Food Nutr Sci 3:621–626

Saharan K, Khetarpaul N (1994) Protein quality traits of vegetable and field peas: varietal differences. Plant Foods Hum Nutr 45:11–22

Salunkhe DK (ed) (1985) Postharvest biotechnology of food legumes. CRC Press, Boca Raton

San Ireneo MM, Ibanez Sandin MD, Fernandez-Caldas F et al (2000) Specific IgE levels to *Cicer arietinum* (chickpea) in tolerant and non-tolerant children: evaluation of boiled and raw extracts. Int Arch Allergy Immunol 121:137–143

Sangdhu KS, Lim ST (2008) Digestibility of legume starches as influenced by its physical and structural properties. Carbohydr Polym 71:245–252

Sanjeewa WGT, Wanasundara JPD, Pietrasik Z et al (2010) Characterization of chickpea (*Cicer arietinum* L.) flours and application in low-fat pork bologna as a model system. Food Res Int 43:617–626

Satterlee LD, Bembers M, Kendrick JG (1975) Functional properties of the great northern bean (*Phaseolus vulgaris*) protein isolates. J Food Sci 40:81–84

Siegel A, Fawcett B (1976) Food legume processing and utilization. International Development Research Centre (IDRC), Ottawa

Silva-Cristobal L, Osorio-Diaz P, Tovar J et al (2010) Chemical composition, carbohydrate digestibility, and antioxidant capacity of cooked black bean, chickpea, and lentil Mexican varieties. CyTA J Food 8:7–14

Simons CW, Hall C III (2018) Consumer acceptability of gluten-free cookies containing raw cooked and germinated pinto bean flours. Food Sci Nutr 6:77–84

Simons CW, Hall C III, Tulbek M et al (2015) Acceptability and characterization of extruded pinto, navy and black beans. J Sci Food Agric 95:2287–2291

Singhal A, Karaca AC, Tyler R et al (2016) Pulse proteins: from processing to structure-function relationships. In: Grain legumes. InTech. https://doi.org/10.5772/64020

Snauwaert F, Markakis P (1976) Effect of germination and gamma irradiation on the oligosaccharides of navy beans (*Phaseolus vulgaris* L.). Lebensm Wiss U-Technol 9:93–95

Sosulski FW, Wu KK (1988) High-fiber breads containing field pea hulls, wheat, corn, and wild oat brans. Cereal Chem 65:186–191

Sosulski FW, Youngs C (1979) Yield and functional properties of air-classified protein and starch fractions from eight legume flours. J Am Oil Chem Soc 56:292–295

Spink PS, Zabik ME, Uebersax MA (1984) Dry-roasted air-classified edible bean protein flour use in cake doughnuts. Cereal Chem 61:251–254

Sun XD, Arntfield SD (2010) Gelation properties of salt-extracted pea protein induced by heat treatment. Food Res Int 43:509–515

Tiwari BK, Singh N (2012) Pulse Chemistry and Technology. RSC Publishing, Cambridge UK pp 107–133

Tudorica CM, Kuri V, Brennan CS (2002) Nutritional and physicochemical characteristics of dietary fiber enriched pasta. J Agric Food Chem 50:347–356

Tyler RT (1984) Impact milling quality of grain legumes. J Food Sci 49:925–930

Tyler RT, Youngs CG, Sosulski FW (1981) Air classification of legumes. I. Separation efficiency, yield, and composition of the starch and protein fractions. Cereal Chem 58:144–148

U.S. Department of Agriculture (2012) Agricultural Research Service. USDA National Nutrient Database for Standard Reference, release 25. http://www.ars.usda.gov/ba/bhnrc/ndl. Accessed 30 Nov 2017

Utrilla-Coello RG, Osorio-Díaz P, Bello-Pérez LA (2007) Alternative use of chickpea flour in breadmaking: chemical composition and starch digestibility of bread. Food Sci Technol Int 13:323–327

Verma MM, Ledward DA, Lawrie RA (1984) Utilization of chickpea flour in sausages. Meat Sci 11:109–121

Vidal-Valverde C, Frias J, Estrella I et al (1994) Effect of processing on some antinutritional factors of lentils. J Agric Food Chem 42:2291–2295

Vose JR, Basterrechea MJ, Gorin PAJ et al (1976) Air classification of field peas and horsebean flours: chemical studies of starch and protein fractions. Cereal Chem 53:928–936

Wang N, Daun J (2004) Effect of variety and crude protein content on nutrients and certain anti-nutrients in field peas (*Pisum sativium*). J Sci Food Agric 84:1021–1029

Wang N, Daun J (2006) Effect of variety and crude protein content on nutrients and certain anti-nutrients in lentils (*Lens culinaris*). Food Chem 95:493–502

Wang J, Rosella CM, de Barber CB (2002) Effect of the addition of different fibres on wheat dough performance and bread quality. Food Chem 79:221–226

Wang N, Daun JK, Malcolmson LJ (2003) Relationship between physicochemical and cooking properties, and effects of cooking on antinutrients, of yellow field peas (*Pisum sativum*). J Sci Food Agric 83:1228–1237

Wang N, Hatcher DW, Toews R et al (2009) Influence of cooking and dehulling on nutritional composition of several varieties of lentils (*Lens culinaris*). LWT Food Sci Tech 42:842–848

Wang N, Hatcher DW, Tyler RT et al (2010) Effect of cooking on the composition of beans (*Phaseolus vulgaris* L.) and chickpeas (*Cicer arietinum*). Food Res Int 43:589–594

Youngs CG (1975) Primary processing of pulse. In: Harapiak JT (ed) Oilseeds and pulse crops in western Canada – a symposium. Western Co-operative Fertilizers Ltd., Calgary

Zare F, Boye JI, Orsat V et al (2011) Microbial, physical and sensory properties of yogurt supplemented with lentil flour. Food Res Int 44:2482–2488

Zare F, Orsat V, Boye JI (2015) Functional, physical and sensory properties of pulse ingredients incorporated into orange and apple juice beverages. J Food Res 4:143–156

Zhao YH, Manthey FA, Chang SKC et al (2005) Quality characteristics of spaghetti as affected by green and yellow pea, lentil, and chickpea flours. J Food Sci 70:s371–s376

Zucco F, Borsuk Y, Arntfield SD (2011) Physical and nutritional evaluation of wheat cookies supplemented with pulse flours of different particle sizes. LWT Food Sci Tech 44:2070–2076

# Index

Printed in the United States
By Bookmasters